Clinica

OTOLARYNGOLOGY

Clinical Cases in
OTOLARYNGOLOGY

Nirmal Kumar Soni
MBBS MS (ENT)
Honorary Professor and Head
Department of ENT
Rajasthan University of Health Sciences
Jaipur, Rajasthan, India

Ex-Professor and Head
Department of ENT
Sardar Patel Medical College and
Associate Group of PBM Hospitals
Bikaner, Rajasthan, India

Co-author
Lokesh Kumar Bhama
MBBS DLO (ENT) Clinical Ordinature
Senior Consultant
Department of ENT
Balaji Hospital and Research Center
Bikaner, Rajasthan, India

Foreword
Raja Babu Panwar

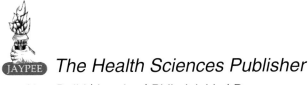

The Health Sciences Publisher
New Delhi | London | Philadelphia | Panama

Jaypee Brothers Medical Publishers (P) Ltd

Headquarters
Jaypee Brothers Medical Publishers (P) Ltd
4838/24, Ansari Road, Daryaganj
New Delhi 110 002, India
Phone: +91-11-43574357
Fax: +91-11-43574314
Email: jaypee@jaypeebrothers.com

Overseas Offices

J.P. Medical Ltd
83 Victoria Street, London
SW1H 0HW (UK)
Phone: +44 20 3170 8910
Fax: +44 (0)20 3008 6180
Email: info@jpmedpub.com

Jaypee Medical Inc
325 Chestnut Street
Suite 412, Philadelphia, PA 19106, USA
Phone: +1 267-519-9789
Email: support@jpmedus.com

Jaypee Brothers Medical Publishers (P) Ltd
Bhotahity, Kathmandu
Nepal
Phone: +977-9741283608
Email: kathmandu@jaypeebrothers.com

Jaypee-Highlights Medical Publishers Inc
City of Knowledge, Bld. 237, Clayton
Panama City, Panama
Phone: +1 507-301-0496
Fax: +1 507-301-0499
Email: cservice@jphmedical.com

Jaypee Brothers Medical Publishers (P) Ltd
17/1-B Babar Road, Block-B, Shaymali
Mohammadpur, Dhaka-1207
Bangladesh
Mobile: +08801912003485
Email: jaypeedhaka@gmail.com

Website: www.jaypeebrothers.com
Website: www.jaypeedigital.com

Clinical Cases in Otolaryngology

First Edition: **2016**

ISBN: 978-93-85891-61-8

Printed at Sanat Printers

Dedicated to

My parents—Bhim Raj Soni and Krishna Devi Soni
who are my center of inspiration and whatever I could achieved
are due to their blessing.
Most specially to my beloved wife—Shrikanta Soni
a wonderful partner, friend, a smartest internist
a role model of mother to serve her children
and well-trained family manager!

Nirmal Kumar Soni

FOREWORD

Most aspiring ENT teacher, surgeon and academician on preparing a book dealing for clinical cases by developing his own approaches is praise worthy. This book is written in a practical manner concise with questions and answers of problems at every step of the disease process without compromising the coverage of the subject. The book, *Clinical Cases in Otolaryngology* is simple, lucid and an easily understandable for undergraduates, postgraduates and general practitioners. Dr Nirmal Kumar Soni has made all possible efforts to give clinical pictures of all routinely encountered cases in ENT practice. I wish him all the best for this book which will become a major footing stone in ENT literature and probably best used as a basis for practical approach to clinical ENT case study.

Raja Babu Panwar
MD DNB (Cardio)
Vice-Chancellor
Rajasthan University of Health Sciences
Jaipur, Rajasthan, India

PREFACE

The spectrum of otorhinolaryngology and head and neck surgery is rapidly and vastly expending with the introduction of recent minimal invasive and noninvasive diagnostic and consequent therapeutic advancement.

As a result there is rapid expansion of descriptive aspect of the various disorders of the ENT region. There are numerous books on ENT and head & neck surgery which cover almost all the theoretical aspects of the subject but these texts do not solve all the problems which arise during clinical case study, in practical approach to diagnosis and subsequent management aspect of the disease.

During my 40 years journey through my teaching experience of ENT and head & neck surgery to undergraduates and postgraduates, I came across the problem faced by the students who are keen to learn the subject in easy and simple manner. To get this practical clinical knowledge for case study, the students have to plod through several books within a short span of time and consequently, they fail to assimilate the subject satisfactorily.

Due to this problem of the students, learning physicians and my experience with the ever-rising problems, I was prompted to write the present book. This endure would assist its readers in finding a perspective not always easily available from the standard textbooks.

Now the field of ENT and head & neck surgery being inconceivably vast, "what to study?" "how to study" and "how to face the problem" of the clinical cases during examination and also during day-to-day practice is a problem faced by the students and clinicians. This book will serve a good solution by providing easy answer to these perplexing questions, so that the reader can readily grasp the subject which is very useful in qualifying examination as well as in their practical field of training.

The clinical case presentation, etiopathology, salient features, relevant investigative procedures, differential diagnosis and principle of treatment of surgical problems of the different ENT cases have been lucidly and thoroughly discussed.

To make the book useful, easily understandable and graspable, I have tried to put clinical pictures of almost all cases which were available in my collection of clinical practice of about 40 years.

Despite best efforts, some errors might have crept in, constrictive criticism and valuable suggestions for improvement of book will be most welcome.

I tried my best to utilize the academic experience of publishing about 200 research papers on ENT subjects in various international and national reputed journals, in preparation of the matter in the present book with the aim that it will be useful as clinical aid to students in cultivation of the art of clinical diagnosis.

Nirmal Kumar Soni

ACKNOWLEDGMENTS

First and foremost I am obliged to my great teacher *Late* Professor Dr P Chatterji under whose guidance and constant prodding, I learned the art of otolaryngology and cervicofacial surgery and established my career as a teacher, academician and a practitioner. I am grateful to my teacher Dr DL Chhangani, who initiated and grew my interest in subject during embryonic phase of my postgraduation in the ENT and subsequently he encouraged me to rise at every step in academic as well as other phases of my life.

Dr Manoj Bhama, an Orthopedic Surgeon, my elder son who really pushed me in this venture and sincerely contributed for this project must be acknowledged here. I am thankful to his wife Mrs Meenakshi Johari Bhama, for her outrightly support in this endeavor.

Dr Lokesh Kumar Bhama, an ENT Surgeon, my younger son deserve special thanks, who help me at every step in preparation of this book, as a co-author. I am thankful to his wife Mrs Archana Varma Bhama, for her continuous assistance through in this work.

Moreover, I am thankful to my affectionate daughter Suman Bhama Soni, and her husband Sunil Soni, for useful contribution in this regard. I should not forget to thank my grandsons (Potra) Dhruv, Nikhil, Shourya and Shivang (Dohita) and Reshu (Dohiti) for extraordinary lovely cooperation.

All the members of my Soni Bhama family specially Prakash Chand, Niranjan Kumar, Shri Ram and Prem Chand also deserve acknowledgement for extending their help and blessing in preparation of the present book.

I am thankful to my colleagues Dr AS Rathore, Dr JP Gupta, Dr Deep Chand, Dr HM Sharma who worked in ENT Department, Sardar Patel Medical College with me like friends and always encouraged me for academic activities, writing the manuscripts and publishing papers, and helped me to reach at the present status.

I thank my office assistant Mr Rahul Parihar, for typing the manuscript and my clinic assistant Mr Ramavatar, for invisible help.

Last but not least, I am greatly indebted to Shri Jitendar P Vij (Group Chairman), Mr Ankit Vij (Group President) and Mr Tarun Duneja (Director-Publishing) of M/s Jaypee Brothers Medical Publishers (P) Ltd, New Delhi, India, for their sincere efforts and constant cooperation for which the publication of this book has become a reality.

Nirmal Kumar Soni

CONTENTS

SECTION 1: Diseases of the Ear

SECTION 2: Head and Neck Diseases from ENT Perspective

SECTION 3: Diseases of Throat
(Oral Cavity, Pharynx and Larynx)

SECTION 4: Diseases of the Nose and Sinuses

SECTION 1

Diseases of the Ear

Microtia

CASE: A malformed small-sized pinna.

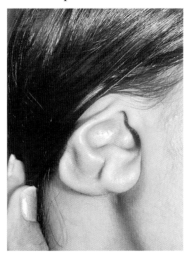

Fig.1: Microtia (right)

Provisional Diagnosis: Microtia

Q.1 How does a malformed pinna develop?
Ans. The auricle develops from the six hillocks of His. Maldevelopment or failure of fusion can result in gross abnormalities of the ear. Microtia is a deformed small-sized pinna (Fig. 1). It may or may not be associated with middle or inner ear abnormalities.

Q.2 What is the classification of congenital malformed pinna?
Ans. 1. Grade I: Normal ear.
  2. Grade II: All pinna elements present but malformed.
  3. Grade III: Rudementary bar only.
  4. Grade IV: Absent pinna (Anotia).

Q.3 What are the investigations to be done in malformed pinna?

Ans. 1. Documenting the defect.
     2. Examining the external auditory canal (for associated abnormalities).
     3. Hearing assessment.
     4. CT scan (to assess middle ear, ossicles or cochlear anatomy).

Q.4 What is the treatment?

Ans. The treatment depends on type and severity of abnormalities:
     1. Minor abnormalities (grade II): No treatment is required.
     2. Major deformity (grades III and IV anotia):
         – Removal of rudimentary pinna
         – Bone anchored hearing aid (BAHA)
         – Abutment to attach an artificial pinna
         – Plastic reconstruction of pinna (if possible).

Preauricular Sinus

CASE: A small dimple or punctum anterior to the tragus.

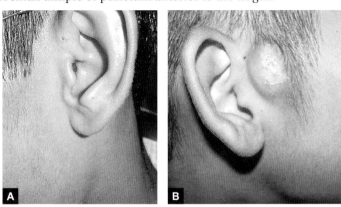

Figs 1A and B: (A) Preauricular sinus; (B) Infected preauricular sinus as an abscess

Provisional Diagnosis: Preauricular Sinus

Q.1 What is preauricular sinus?
Ans. A congenital sinus in front of the pinna since birth and is caused by incomplete fusion of the hillocks of His (between Ist and IInd branchial arches).

Q.2 What is embryological basis of preauricular sinus?
Ans. The pinna develops from fusion of six tubercles (tragus, crus helix, antihelixes, antitragus's and ear lobule) surrounding the external auditory canal. Failure of fusion of anterior tubercles results into one or more narrow blind pits. Most commonly due to failure of fusion between tubercle one and two. The pit sometimes continue deep to form a sinus (Fig. 1A). If the sinus is occluded, a cyst is formed.

Q.3 What is usual site of preauricular sinus?
Ans. It is between the tragus and the crus helix.

Q.4 What is the direction of tract of preauricular sinus?
Ans. It is downwards and forwards.

Q.5 What are different presenting features of preauricular sinus?

Ans. 1. A pit in front of the ear, unilateral or bilateral (frequently one of the parents has similar pits).
2. Whitish discharge from sinus opening.
3. Recurrent abscess with nonhealing infected sinus in front of the ear (Fig. 1B).
4. Persistent preauricular ulcer.

Q.6 What are the differential diagnosis of preauricular sinus?

Ans. 1. Post-traumatic preauricular sinus.
2. Tuberculous sinus (due to preauricular lymph node).
3. Sinus as a result of infected or incised preauricular dermoid cyst.

Q.7 What is treatment of preauricular sinus?

Ans. Treatment depends on presenting features.
1. A symptomatic sinus: Usually no treatment except advice for local hygiene to prevent infection.
2. Presentation as abscess or infected sinus.
   a. Incision and drainage by vertical incision.
   b. Complete excision (after 3–6 weeks later) of entire sinus and its ramification. Sinus can be delineated by injecting methylene blue with hydrogen peroxide in the sinus tract.
3. Presensation with an area of ramifying epithelium lined tract in preauricular region: Treated by wide excision of the involved skin and subcutaneous tissue preserving the facial nerve.

Preauricular Appendages (Accessory Auricular Tags)

CASE: Patient presents with small nodular like swelling or tag in front of the ear.

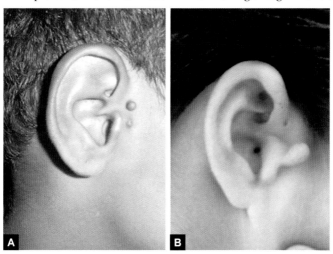

Figs 1A and B: (A) Preauricular tag and accessory auricle; (B) Preauricular tag

Provisional Diagnosis: Preauricular Appendages

Q.1 What are preauricular appendages?

Ans. These are covered tags (Fig. 1B) that appears on a line drawn from the tragus to the angle of mouth, present since birth. They may contain small pieces of cartilage (separated from the pinna).

Q.2 What are the differential diagnosis?

Ans. 1. An enlarged preauricular lymph node.
  2. A parotid gland tumor.

Q.3 What is the treatment?

Ans. Excision from cosmetic point of view.

Q.4 What is tag and accessory auricle?

Ans. Small masses composed of skin and fat only, is skin tags (Fig. 1B). When it contains cartilage in addition, it is called accessory auricle (Fig. 1A).

Cauliflower Ear

CASE: A typical disfigured deformity of the shape of the auricle.

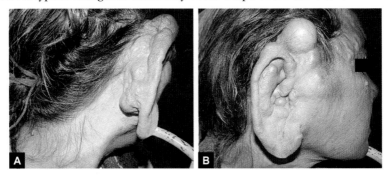

Figs 1A and B: Disfigured auricle like cauliflower ear

Provisional Diagnosis: Cauliflower Ear

Q.1 What is cauliflower ear?

Ans. It is a disfigured deformity of the auricle as a result of organization of extravasated blood clot and fibrosis with cartilage loss (due to pressure necrosis of the cartilage) in a hematoma of the auricle (Figs 1A and B).

Q.2 How is it formed?

Ans. There is collection of blood between the perichondrium and cartilage due to trauma (boxing and wrestling) which leads to pressure necrosis of the cartilage. Subsequent infection, organization of extravasated blood clot, and fibrosis with cartilage loss, leads to the typical deformity "cauliflower ear".

Q.3 What are the features of cauliflower ear?

Ans. 1. Disfigured pinna.
2. Sometimes fluctuant and sometimes firm swelling fixed to the cartilage of the ear filling the hollows of the pinna.

Q.4 What are the complications of cauliflower ear?

Ans. 1. Perichondritis.

     2. Deformity of pinna.

Q.5 How can it be prevented?

Ans. It is a complication of hematoma of the ear. Hematoma should be treated properly.

     1. Prophylactic heavy dose of broad-spectrum antibiotics.

     2. Aspiration is usually difficult due to the thickness of the clot.

     3. Incision and removal of clot. Suturing may be done, if large incision has been made. Pressure bandage is applied for about 5 days to prevent reaccumulation.

CASE

5

Keloid Ear Lobule

CASE: A firm smooth spherical sessile nodule behind the ear lobule. History of ear piercing and subsequent itching.

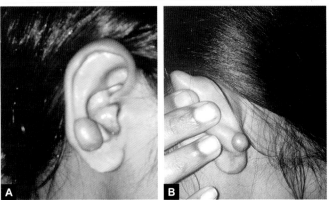

Figs 1A and B: Keloid pinna after ear piercing

Provisional Diagnosis: Keloid

Q.1 What is keloid?
Ans. Keloid means claw like. It is a hypertrophied scar with claw-like extension into the adjoining tissue.

Q.2 What are the points in favor of diagnosis?
Ans. There are several points like:
1. History of ear piercing
2. Complaint of itching
3. The swelling is firm, smooth with claw-like progressives in all side upwards (Figs A and B).

Q.3 What are the types of keloid?
Ans. Keloids are of two types:
1. Spontaneous: It is commonly seen in front of the chest as a butterfly like swelling.
2. Acquired: It is seen at the site of pinprick, incisional scar, burn, and abscess.

Q.4 What is differences between keloid and hypertrophied scar?

Ans. There are several differences:

Hypertrophied scar	Keloid
1. Always on a scar	1. It can develop on scar or even spontaneously.
2. Scar does not become progressive even after 6 months	2. It become progressive after 6 months.
3. Smooth edge, claw like process are not seen.	3. Irregular edge with claw-like progressive from sides at lesion.
4. Does not invade adjoining normal tissue.	4. Invades adjoining normal tissue.
5. Itching is usually absent.	5. Persistent itching.
6. Swelling is white to pale.	6. Swelling is pinkish and red, more at margin.
7. No recurrence after excision.	7. Recurrent after excision commonly.
8. Microscopically, it consists of mature fibrous tissue without any blood vessels.	8. It consists of immature fibroblasts with immature blood vessels.
9. Smooth surface	9. Lobulated or coarsely irregular.
10. Local temperature normal.	10. Warm to touch.
11. Firm, thick and nontender.	11. Harder and tender.

Q.5 What are the complications of keloid?

Ans. 1. It may get infected.
   2. May under go malignant changes (Marjolin's ulcer).
   3. Recurs following excision.

Q.6 What is the etiology of keloid?

Ans. Definte etiology is not known. Several factors are:
   1. Familial conditions.
   2. Dark skin people are more prone.
   3. Patients with tuberculosis are affected more.
   4. Scars opposite to Langer's line are affected more.

Q.7 Describe the line of treatment?

Ans. Excision is almost always followed by recurrence, so conservation treatment may be tried.
   1. Intrakeloid injection of hydrocortisone, hyaluronidase or vitamin A.
   2. Ultrasonic therapy.
   3. Radiotherapy.
   4. Laser beam therapy.
   5. Intrakeloid excision with skin grafting.

CASE

6

Exostoses
(Diaphyseal Aclasis)

CASE: Multiple painless nodular swellings in the lumen of external auditory canal (both ears).

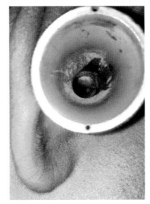

Fig. 1: Exostoses

Provisional Diagnosis: Exostoses (Surfer's Ear)

Q.1. What is exostosis?

Ans. These are periosteal outgrowths, which grow away from the ivory bone so called exostoses. These usually occur at epiphysis of growing end of bone (Fig. 1).

Q.2 Is it a bony tumor?

Ans. It is considered as cancellous osteoma but actually it is a disorder of bone growth and is, not a tumor. It is cancellous bone covered with cortical bone. Base is broad and other end is covered with cartilage.

Q.3 What are the points in favor of dignosis of exostoses?

Ans. The points are:
1. Painless and hard bony swelling in the external ear canal.
2. It is a fixed to bone having smooth surface. These are multiple and usually bilateral.

Q.4 What are the other salient features?

Ans. 1. It is common in persons with multiple exposure to swimming in cold water.
   2. It is painless, slow growing bony swelling.
   3. It has smooth surface and can be multiple.
   4. Swelling is adherent to underlying bone with broad base.
   5. It is mainly found in cartilaginous bone.

Q.5 What is the finding in X-rays?

Ans. It is seen as a bony swelling from the surface of canal as an outgrowth.

Q.6 What are the complications of exostoses?

Ans. There are:
   1. Infection.
   2. Deafness due to occlusion of canal.
   3. Impacted wax and desquamated epithelial debris—due to defective cleaning mechanism.

Q.7 What is the treatment of exostoses?

Ans. Excision of exostoses with micro-drill.

Osteoma

CASE: A localized smooth, slow-growing bony swelling at the postauricular region.

Provisional Diagnosis: Osteoma

Q.1 What is osteoma?
Ans. Osteoma is a benign tumor of cortical bone.

Q.2 What are the types of osteoma?
Ans. There are two types osteoma, these are:
1. Concellous type—appears as projection, pedunculated like mushrooms, arises from metaphysial surface of bone.
2. Compact type (Ivory osteoma)—is ivory hard, sessile, dome-shaped painless swelling with well-defined edge and is seft-limiting over the skull and facial bones.

Q.3 What are complications of osteoma?
Ans. Complications are:
1. Deformity.
2. Pressure symptoms.
3. Focal epilepsy (if it arises from inner table of the facial or skull bone).

Q.4 What is treatment of osteoma?
Ans. No treatment is usually required if it is asymptomatic. The tumor is excised for cosmetic purpose. Excision is done by chiseling across the base.

Q.5 What are common sites for compact osteoma?
Ans. It occurs in skull, orbit, paranasal sinuses, mastoid, external auditory canal and jaw bone. It is common in frontal sinus in temporal bone, and in mastoid region.

Q.6 What is the finding in X-ray?
Ans. On X-ray, it shows sessile opacity of excessive dense bone (more whiter or denser than the bone) with a well-circumscribed edge.

8

Otomycosis
(Otomycotic Disease)

CASE: A patient presents with itching and mild discharge in the ear. Otoscopy reveals a wet news-paper like debris in the deeper part of external auditory canal.

Provisional Diagnosis: Otomycosis

Q.1 What are the predisposing factors for otomycosis?
Ans. 1. Rainy season and humidity.
   2. Moisture—water borne—swimming and bath.
   3. Antibiotics—broad spectrum and prolonged use.
   4. Steroids—prolonged use, systematic or local.
   5. Diabetes.
   6. Pregnancy.
   7. Chronic suppurative otitis media (CSOM).
   8. Operated wide mastoid cavity.
   9. AIDS and immuno-compromised person.
   10. Hot and humid climate.
   11. Persons wearing hearing aid.

Q.2 What are causative agents of otomycosis?
Ans. 1. *Asparagillus*: Niger (black), alba (white), fumigatous (gray)
   2. Candida (Monilial): *Candida albicans*
   3. Other: *Dermatophytes*.

Q.3 What are main symptoms?
Ans. These are:
   1. Itching—Most common and prominent symptom.
   2. Sense of fullness.
   3. Deafness—Due to collection of moist debris in the canal.
   4. Pain—As deeper tissue becomes inflamed.
   5. Discharge—If secondary infection.
   6. Tinnitus—May be present.

Q.4 What are different features of otomycosis?

Ans. Various findings can be:

1. Cotton wool like mass in the ear canal.
2. Wet newspaper like mass—presenting multicolor appearance ranging from white to gray, brown or black color or putaceous material.
3. Wet bloating paper like debris mass of grayish white color.
4. Conidiophore of *Aspergillus niger*—may be seen as black specks in the debris (Fig. 1).
5. A mass of fine filaments projecting from meatal wall.

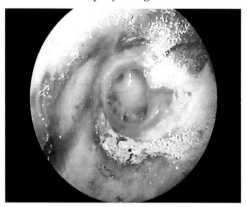

Fig. 1: Otomycosis with spores in the external auditory canal

Q.5 Can otomycosis exist without any positive finding?

Ans. Yes, no sign. If a case of otitis externa fails to response to treatment, possibly of fungus.

Q.6 How is dignosis confirmed?

Ans. Diagnosis is confirmed:

1. By clinical criteria.
2. By microscopic examination of debris.
3. By culture.

Q.7 What is treatment of otomycosis?

Ans. Ear toilet and cleaning:

1. By suction, mopping or syringing.
2. Antifungal drops like clotrimazole, tolnaftate, micronizole, nystatin, hamysin.
3. Antifungal antiseptics like gention violet (1%), alcohal and spirit, mercurochrome.
4. Keratolytic agent: like salicylic acid 1% in spirit.
5. Systemic: (a) Antibiotics—to control secondary infection; (b) Antihistaminics—as antipruritic; (c) Analgesics; (d) Antifungal (orally) in resistant cases.

Q.8 In which part of the ear otomycosis is common?

Ans. 1. In the deeper part (bony part) of external canal.
2. Mastoid cavity (operated and wide).

Traumatic Perforations of the Tympanic Membrane

CASE: A large oval shaped perforation in anterior inferior quadrant with red and ragged margin and zone of ecchymosis. There is history of slap on the ear.

Provisional Diagnosis: Traumatic Perforation of Tympanic Membrane

Q.1 What are common causes of traumatic perforation?
Ans. It occurs due to either:
1. Direct violence.
2. Indirect violence or injury.

Q.2 What are causes of direct injury leading to perforation of TM?
Ans. Direct violence like:
1. Attempt to clean the ear or to remove foreign body (FB), or to relieve the itching (self injury) by matchsticks, hair pins or any sharp objects.
2. Itrogenic: By forceful syringing, attempt to remove the FB, Eustachian catheterization, erroneously applying caustic or acidic solution in place of ear drops.
3. Physiological: Sneezing or forceful Valsalva procedure.

Q.3 What are the causes of perforation of TM due to indirect violence?
Ans. These are:
1. Strong slap.
2. Blast injury (exposure to violent explosion or bomb blast).
3. Fracture of base of skull (hematoma).
4. Trauma to mandible.
5. Barotrauma—rapid descent during air travel.

Q.4 What are common symptoms in traumatic perforation?
Ans. Various symptoms are:
1. Pain: It may be severe, sometimes patient may faint, occaisnally pain may be absent (in case of rupture of thin tympanic membrane).
2. Hearing loss: Present but may pass unnoticed because of normal second ear.
3. Tinnitus.

4. Giddiness: It may occur in blast injury.

5. Bleeding from ear: It occurs in case of direct trauma.

Q.5 What are signs of perforation of TM by direct trauma?

Ans. 1. Perforation: Usually in the lower part or in the posterosuperior part of TM (most superficial part)

2. Perforation: Linear tear.

3. Perforation has ecchymotic zone on the margin (extravasation of blood).

4. The size and shape resembles the object which caused it.

Q.6 What are findings in perforation caused by indirect violence?

Ans. 1. In slap or blast injury: The perforation has ragged edges or punched out margin (Figs 1A and B).

2. Margin is red with hyperemia.

3. Usually large slit or oval in shape.

4. Usually in anteroinferior quadrant.

5. Injury may be due to inner ear: Causing either concussion or hemorrage in the labyrinth (leading to giddiness, marked and permanent deafness).

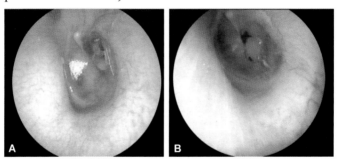

Figs 1A and B: Otoscopic views of traumatic perforation of tympanic membrane

Q.7 What are pecularities of blast injury?

Ans. Bomb blast may cause: (a) A large perforation; (b) Two perforations, (c) Perforation of both ear; (d) No perforation but damage the inner ear leading to vertigo and sensorineural hearing loss.

Q.8 Can the tympanic membrane heal after perforation?

Ans. Perforation of TM usually heals. Healing occurs by migration of epithelium from umbo towards periphery, at the rate of 0.05 mm per day.

Q.9 How dose the tympanic membrane heal?

Ans. The outer epithelial (skin) and inner endothelial (mucosal) layer regenrate to seal the perforation, but middle fibrous (mesothelial) layer dose not regenerate. Newly fromed two layered membrane is called monometric membrane and it is usually transparent.

Q.10 What investigations are required?

Ans. 1. Tuning fork tests: Conductive hearing loss.
   2. Audiometry (pure tone): Mostly conductive hearing loss, mixed deafness when cochlea is damaged in blast injury.
   3. BERA: Indicated in malignerer and functional and noncooperative medicolegal cases.

Q.11 What is the treatment of traumatic perforation of TM?

Ans. 1. Nothing in the ear, avoid water in the ear.
   2. Sterilized cotton in meatus.
   3. Nasal decongestant.
   4. Prophylactic antibiotics.
   5. Healing to perforation occurs in most cases in 6–8 weeks.
   6. Unhealed perforation: It may require mayringoplasty.
   7. Reposition of indrawn ragged margin of perforation under microscope and paper patching.

Q.12 What is paper patch of TM (paperplasty)?

Ans. 1. A patch of paper (cut circular piece of cigarette or rice paper) is applied on the TM which act as scaffold for reepithelialization process, in small or moderate size perforation, which does not heal spontaneously.
   2. In chronic perforation or central perforation of CSOM, the margin of the perforation is made raw or abraded by chemical caity (silver nitrate)or by surgical removel of edge rim before applying paper patch.
   3. Patient is followed up and reviewed monthly. If required, the procedure may be repeated.

CASE

10

Secretory Otitis Media

CASE: A 10 year-old child presented with deafness in both ear. Otoscopy reveals lustreless TM with fluid level (hairline) and air bubbles in one ear while the other ear shows evidence of retraction.

Provisional Diagnosis: Secretory Otitis Media

Q. 1 What is secretory otitis media (SOM)?
Ans. Chronic inflammatory changes in the mucous lining of middle ear with formation of sterile effusion.

Q. 2 What are other name of secretory otitis media?
Ans. Several names are nonsuppurative otitis media, glue ear, serous otitis media, mucoid otitis media, exudative otitis media, catarrhal otitis media, middle ear effusion.

Q. 3 What are main epidemiological features?
Ans. It is common in western and developed countries. It is more frequent in children than adults. In children both ears are affected. Prevalence is 3–4% of all ENT diseases and it occurs more commonly in young school children.

Q. 4 What are various etiological factors?
Ans. Several factors responsible are
1. Anatomical: DNS, cleft palate, other abnormalities of hard and soft palate, oral SMF, fibrosis of palate, nasopharyngeal disproportion, craniofacial abnormalities.
2. Physiological: Middle ear gas compositions, allergy, neurovascular and neuroendocrinal factors cause hypersecretion.
3. Pathological: Enlarged tonsil, adenoids, polyp, rhinitis, sinusitis, nasopharyngitis, nasopharyngeal tumor.
4. Itrogenic: Inadequate antibiotic, undrained and unresolved otitis media.
5. Geographical factors: Common in western countries, uncommon in tropical countries
6. General diseases: Hypogammaglobulinemia, AIDS, hypothyroidism, normal disturbances of mucociliary transport system, immunological factors.
7. Social factors: Passive smoker, propping a bottle in a supine infant's mouth (bottle feeding in supine position).

Q. 5 Secretory otitis media occurs commonly in cleft palate. Why?

Ans. 1. Chronic nasopharyngitis and Eustachian tube infection.
2. Palate muscles less effective in opening Eustachian tube.

Q. 6 What are reasons of not improving SOM following cleft palate surgery?

Ans. 1. Damage to nerve supply of muscles during dissection.
2. Fracture of the hammulus during repair to release tendon of medial part of tensor palati muscle.
3. Postoperative scarring interfere with muscular function controlling patency of Eustachian tube.

Q. 7 What are pathogenesis of middle ear effusion?

Ans. 1. Either failure of ventilation of middle ear or drain of middle ear due to Eustachian tube obstruction.
   Causes are:
   i. Nlarged adenoids
   ii. Chronic rhinosinusitis
   iii. Chronic tonsillitis
   iv. Tumors of nasopharynx
   v. Palatal defects—cleft palate, fibrosis, oral SMF, paralysis of palate
   vi. Allergy—mucosal edema
   vii. Unresolved otitis media—inadequate antibiotic and diminished resistance.
2. Increased secretory activity in the middle ear:
   i. Allergy
   ii. Postotitis media
   iii. Viral infection, e.g. respiratory syncytial virus, adenovirus.

Q. 8 What are the characteristics of fluid in secretory otitis media?

Ans. The fluid may be serous, seromucoid, seropurulent, mucoid, mucopurulent, with glue-like consistency. Color of fluid may be clear, opaque, yellow or dark brown.

Q. 9 What are various symptoms of secretory otitis media?

Ans. 1. Asymptomatic: It may be quite incidious.
2. Deafness: Usually the presenting and sometime the only symptom, incidious in onset, mild to moderate degree, sometime fluctuating, usually worse with cold.
3. Autophony: Patient listens his own voice in his own ears.
4. Earache: Mild pain and discomfort specially in cold.
5. Sensation of fluid: Patient may feel as if there is fluid moving in the ear.
6. Delayed or defective speech: Due to deafness specially in young children.
7. Tinnitus: May be presented.
8. Patient is unable to clear the ear by autoinflations.

Q. 10 What are the common signs of secretory otitis media.

Ans. Variable changes in tympanic membrane (TM):

1. Tympanic membrane is often dull, lustreless, opaque with loss of light reflex. Handle of mallius stands out as starkely white against the color change of TM (Fig. 1).

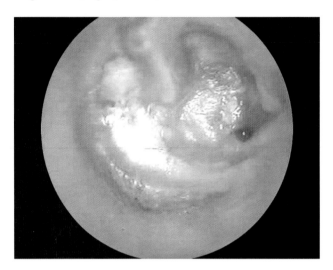

Fig. 1: Otitis media with effusion with tympanosclerotic patches

2. Color of TM: Yellow hue to grayish or bluish or gun-metal.
3. Annular and radiating blood vessels are seen impacted.
4. Retracted TM with diminished mobility.
5. Bulging of posterior part of TM.
6. Fluid level with air bubbles: If fluid is thin and TM is transparent.
7. Fluid level with horizontally crecentic hairline.
8. Full bulging of TM.
9. Collapse of pars flaccida or posterior part of pars tensa or both these together.
10. Complete collapse of whole drum head.
11. Thinning of collapse membrane.
12. Blue drum—bluish in color.
13. Gunmetal appearance of TM.
14. On siegelization—there is characteristic snap back of TM due to the surface tension of the fluid during release of suction.
15. Pot-belly appearance of TM—fullness in SOM with retracted TM appears to be sagging on lower part.
16. Sago-grain appearance—small spots seen on TM
17. Small pinkish or rossete spots arrange discretely in a coral necklace formation below the umbo of TM is seen in SOM and it occurs in healing viral infection or as a sequel of influenzual myringitis.

Q. 11 What are grades of retraction of pars tensa in SOM?
Ans. Gradation of the retracted pars tensa:
1. Grade I : A slight retraction of TM over annulus
2. Grade II: Tympanic membrane touches the long process of incus
3. Grade III: Tympanic membrane touches the promontory
4. Grade IV: Tympanic membrane adherent to promontory

Q. 12 What are stages of retraction of pars flaccida in SOM?
Ans. 1. Stage I: Slight dimple.
2. Stage II: Pars flaccida retracted maximally and dropped over the neck of malleus.
3. Stage III: As stage II but with erosion of outer attic wall.
4. Stage IV: The retraction is deep and accumulated keratin cannot be reached by suction clearance (Full blown attic retraction pocket).

Q. 13 At what level retraction is called retraction pocket?
Ans. Up to when the floor of retracted sac is seen.

Q. 14 What are the complications and sequelae of SOM?
Ans. These are:
1. Resolution with normal or near normal healing.
2. Adhesive otitis media.
3. CSOM with or without cholesteatoma.
4. Atrophic TM and atelectasis of middle ear.
5. Ossicular necrosis.
6. Tympanic sclerosis.
7. Cholesterol granuloma.

Q. 15 What are the investigations required in SOM?
Ans. 1. Tuning fork tests—show conductive deafness.
2. Audiometry:
   i.   Conductive deafness between 20–40 db
   ii. Rarely there may be associated SNHL due to fluid pressure on round window which disappears on evacuation of fluid.
3. Impedence audiometry:
   i.   Pressure of fluid as indicated by reduced compliance with negative pressure, i.e. flat curve with shift to negative side, i.e. B curve
   ii. Normal external auditory canal volume.
4. X-ray mastoid—may be clouding of air cells due to fluid (lack of air entry)
5. X-ray PNS (Water's view) for sinusitis.
6. X-ray nasopharynx (lateral view) for adenoids.

Q. 16 What are the aims of treatment of SOM?
Ans. 1. Removal of fluid
2. Prevention of its recurrence by treating predisposing factors like adenoids, DNS, tonsil, allergy, etc.

Q. 17 What is the medical treatment of SOM?
Ans. 1. Nasal decongestant to reduce edema: (i) Oral and (ii) Topical.
2. Antiallergic measures—antihistaminics or steroids.

3. Antibiotics for URI and for unresolved otitis media—β-lactam or amoxicillin or amoxicillin + clavulanic acid for 10–15 days.
4. Middle ear ventilation—Valsalva, politzerization or Eustachian tube catheterization.

Q.18 What are surgical treatments and its indications in SOM?
Ans. 1. Myringotomy and aspiration of fluid in failure cases after at least 3 months of observation.
2. Myringotomy with mucolytic agents, e.g. chymotrypsin or bromhexine or saline instilation before aspiration.
3. Two incisional myringotomy—to aspirate thick glue like secretion "beer can principle" (one in anterosuperior and one in anteroinferior).
4. Urea solution injection into middle ear to liquefy the thick glue has been tried.
5. Grommet insertion—in cases of failure of medical treatment and failure of myringotomy and aspiration (it provides continued ventilation of middle ear). Grommet or tympanotomy tube is left in place for weeks or month or till spontaneous extrusion up to 6 months.

Q. 19 What are the indications of grommet insertion?
Ans. 1. Middle ear effusion of more than 3 months with associated hearing loss of 30 db or more in better ear.
2. Cases with autophony.
3. Chronic retraction pocket of TM.
4. Tympanic atelectasis.
5. Poor response to medical treatment.

Q. 20 How grommet insertion is done?
Ans. Radial incision at 5 o'clock in the anteroinferior quadrant of TM (anterior myringotomy).

Q. 21 How myringotomy is done in SOM?
Ans. An incision is made in anterosuperior or anteroinferior quadrant of T.M. and fluid is aspirated.

Q. 22 Why is anterior myringotomy done in anteroinferior quadrant?
Ans. 1. Secretion is directed towards this quadrant from rest of tympanum.
2. Grommet remains in place longer.
3. More physiological because air normally enter through anterior portion.
4. Secretory cells are more in anterior portion.
5. Less chances of entry of water.

Q. 23 What are complications of grommet insertion?
Ans. Complications are rare laceration of external auditory canal, persistent otorrhea, granuloma formation, cholesteatoma, chronic perforation, TM retraction, flaccidity (segmental weakness), tympanosclerosis, scarring, injury to ossicles.

Q. 24 What other surgical treatment can be done in tractable cases of SOM?

Ans. 1. Tympanotomy—for loculated thick fluid.
   2. Cortical mastoidectomy—rarely in cholesterol granuloma.
   3. Tympanic neurectomy—to decrease the secretion.

Q. 25 What pressure difference is required for locking of Eustachin tube and acute otitic barotrauma and its treatment?

Ans. 1. Pressure difference between the atmosphere and intratympanic is about 60 mm of Hg. Blocking of Eustachian tube occurs during hunt in flying or in diving and decompression. The locking of Eustachian tube can be opened with Valsalva or politzerization but definitely by Eustachian catheterization.
   2. Difference more than 90 mm of Hg on either side of tympanic membrane will result in acute otitic barotrauma which can be treated by Valsalva, antihistaminics and nasal decongestive drops but myringotomy and suction may be needed.

Q. 26 What are criteria for an ideal grommet insertion?

Ans. Criteria for an ideal grommet insertion is as follows:
   1. Easy to insert.
   2. Not get extruded.
   3. Remain patent.
   4. Nonreactive (Inert).

Tympanosclerosis

CASE: White plaques (Chalk patches) present in the tympanic membrane

Provisional Diagnosis: Tympanosclerosis

Q. 1 What is tympanosclerosis?

Ans. It results from healed otitis media due to hyaline degeneration of the fibrous layer of the TM or middle ear mucosa which undergoes calcification and appears like flake of white snow.

Q. 2 What is clinical features?

Ans. White patches on the drum (periphery of TM) and around ossicles, may be asymptomatic or may cause deafness.

Q. 3 What is the treatment of tympanosclerosis?

Ans. 1. Asymptomatic cases—no treatment
   2. Symptomatic cases:
      i.   Excision of patch followed by tympanoplasty and ossiculoplasty
      ii. Stapedectomy
      iii. Hearing aid.

Q. 4 Can tympanosclerosis causes hearing loss?

Ans. 1. A large white plaque may cause conductive hearing loss up to 30 db.
   2. A thick plaque may hamper the mobility of TM.
   3. It may cause adhesion within TM and ossicles.

Chronic Suppurative Otitis Media

CASE: Patient presents with history of nonoffensive, mucopurulent, intermittent ear discharge from the right ear of 6 years duration. He gives history of diminished hearing almost with the same duration from the same ear. He says hearing improves when discharge is present and hearing more impaired when ear is dry. No history of tinnitus, giddiness or pain and bleeding.

Otoscopy reveals kidney-shaped central perforation, medium to large in size, in pars tensa. Visible mucosa of the middle ear is velvety, pinkish and mildly congested. No mastoid tenderness. Tuning-fork tests reveal a moderate conductive deafness.

Provisional Diagnosis: CSOM with Central Perforation (Tubotympanic Disease)

Q.1 What is chronic suppurative otitis media (CSOM) and tubotympanic disease?

Ans. Chronic suppurative otitis media is defined as a long-standing chronic suppurative infection of a part or whole of the middle ear cleft which is characterized by discharge, deafness and a permanent perforation of tympanic membrane.

These are of two types:
1. Tubotympanic or safe or benign type
2. Atticoantral or unsafe or dangerous type.

Tubotympanic disease—is a varient of CSOM in which the disease is confined to mucosa of Eustachian tube and anteroinferior part of the middle ear. It is safe type because there is no danger to the life of the patient, almost in 90% of the cases. About 10% of apparently safe looking ear may be dangerous.

Q.2 Why does patient shows improvement in hearing when ear is wet and discharging?

Ans. In benign perforation with intact ossicular chain, hearing may improve when the discharge covers and closes perforation temporarily. Hearing improves if the round window is covered with secretion due to improved phase difference (shielding effect of round window). In dry ear (Fig. 1) with perforation, sound waves strike both the oval and round windows simultaneously thus cancelling each others effect (cancellation effect).

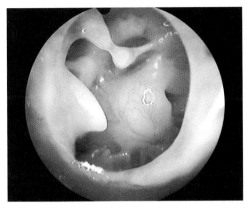

Fig. 1: Provisional diagnosis—chronic suppurative otitis media with tubotympanic disease (safe type)

Q.3 What are the characteristic features of otorrhea in tubotympanic disease?

Ans. Ear discharge is nonoffensive, mucoid, copious in amount, mostly appears at the time of URI or on entry of water in the ear.

Q.4 What are the characteristic features of deafness in tubotympanic disease?

Ans. Hearing loss is conductive type, severity varies from mild to moderate and may rarely exceed 50 db. In long standing case, mixed deafness may be present due to absorption of toxins from the windows. In some cases discharge improves the hearing because of improved phase difference.

Q.5 If earache in tubotympanic disease is present what does it indicates?

Ans. It indicates some form of complications:
1. Acute supervening infection.
2. Anoviated acute otitis externa.
3. Impending dangerous complications like mastoiditis or intracranial complications.

Q.6 What is the significance of bleeding or blood-stained discharge in CSOM?

Ans. It is suggestive of development of granulation or polyp or may suggest dangerous type of perforation.

Q.7 What are the different types of perforations of tympanic membrane (TM) in tubotympanic disease?

Ans. Perforation is central type and always into pars tensa.
    Central perforation—a remnant of TM is present around the margins of perforation.

It can be as follows:
1. Small—pin size to small (less than 25% part of TM).
2. Medium—of different shape round, oval or kidney shape (26–50% part of TM) as shown in Figure 2.
3. Large—kidney shape (51–75% part of TM).
4. Subtotal—perforation extending up to the annulus (more than 75% part of TM).
5. Total—perforation with destruction of annulus.

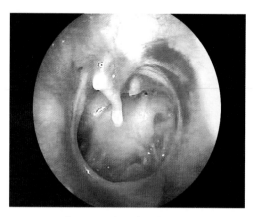

Fig. 2: A subtotal perforation

Q.8 Why a perforation becomes kidney shaped in CSOM?
Ans. Kidney-shaped perforation is due to relatively poor blood supply of the involved area of TM. The blood supply comes from the periphery and travels along the anterior and posterior malleolar folds reaching to handle of malleus. So a kidney-shaped area including the tip of handle of malleus is destroyed.

Q.9 What are etiological factors of tubotympanic disease of CSOM?
Ans. 1. It can be a sequele of acute suppurative otitis media which fails to resolve completely.
  2. Middle-ear infection following acute infections, diseases of childhood, e.g. measles, influenza, diphtheria.
  3. Traumatic large perforation with secondary infection which fails to heal.

Q.10 What are predisposing factors in tubotympanic type of CSOM?
Ans. Predisposing factors in tubotympanic type of CSOM are as follows:
  1. Allergy.
  2. Bathing and swimming in dirty water.
  3. Domestic and economic poor conditions.
  4. Eustachian tube dysfunction.
  5. Low general resistance.
  6. Hereditary predisposing to otorrhea and suppurative affect.
  7. Hypogammaglobulinemia.

8. Infection of tonsils, adenoids and sinuses.
9. Malnutrition.

Q.11 What are the causative organisms in tubotympanic type of CSOM?
Ans. Common causative agents are streptococci, pneumococci or staphylococci. Uncommon are *Bacillus fragilis* and *E. coli.*

Q.12 What are the subtypes of tubotympanic disease?
Ans. 1. Permanent perforation syndrome—central perforation, profuse mucoid or mucopurulent discharge.
2. Persistent mucosal disease which is subdivided into:
    a. Tubal type—in children, mucopurulent discharge, anterior perforation.
    b. Tympanic type—large central perforation, hyperplastic and-oedematous mucosa or even polyp.
    c. Tympanomastoid type—mucosal oedema, purulent, pulsatile discharge in posterosuperior part of tympanum, fetid dischage, granulation.

Q.13 What are the investigations to be done in tubotympanic disease?
Ans. 1. For ear; Pneumonic EARS.
    a. Eustachian tube function for patency.
    b. Audiometry (pure tone)—usually conductive deafness with good air-bone gap.
    c. Radiological—X-ray mastoids both Law's or Owen's or Schuller's view—shows clouding of cells.
    d. Swab for culture and sensitivity of ear discharge—to select proper antibiotics.
2. Routine investigations of:
    a. Blood for Hb, BT, CT, TDLC and blood sugar.
    b. Urine for albumin and sugar.
3. Otomicroscopy—for suction and cleaning for assessment under magnification of the perforation and condition of middle ear mucosa.
4. Paper patch test—to test the integrity of ossicular chain. Audiometry is done to assess the hearing. Paper patch is applied on TM to cover the perforation. Repeated audiometry showed worsening of hearing if ossicular discontinuity is present. Improvement indicates ossicular continuity.

Q.14 What is diffential diagnosis of CSOM?
Ans. 1. Acute otitis media with perforation.
2. Acute necrotising otitis media.
3. Traumatic perforation—has ragged edges.
4. Otitis externa.
5. Secretory otitis media.
6. Tuberculous otitis media.
7. Adhesive otitis media.

Q.15 What are clinical stages in course of the tubobympanic disease?

Ans. There are four clinical stages:

1. Active stage—actively discharging ear.
2. Quiescent stage—not discharging ear but period is less than 3–6 months (Fig. 1).
3. Inactive stage—the ear remains dry for more than 6 months (mucosa is normal).
4. Healed stage—perforation has healed up with or without adhesive changes. Ear is permanently dry.

Q.16 What is treatment in active stage (discharging ear) in tubotympanic disease?

Ans. Treatment is:

1. Aural toilet; dry mopping with cotton swab or by suction.
2. Antibiotics; systemic amoxy+cloxa or ciprofloxacin depending on culture and sensitivity.
3. Aural drops—antibiotics with steroids, ciprofloxacin, ofloxacin, polymyxin, chloramphenicol.
4. Decongestants and antihistaminics.
5. Treatment of predisposing factors like DNS, sinusitis, tonsil, adenoids.
6. General care—keep ear dry, avoid swimming and URI.

Q.17 What is treatment of inactive stage or dry ear in tubotympanic disease?

Ans. Depends on age of the patient and type of perforation;

1. Child and aged person with mild deafness—no surgical treatment is required.
   Otherwise treatment depends on size and site of perforation.
   In perforation less than 5 mm in size—cautry with trichloroacetic acid (20%) or silver nitrate (50%)—is done repeatedly at 7–10 days interval to de-epithelialize margin of perforation and to promote healing.
2. Fat tympanoplasty—if perforation is less than 50% of the TM.
3. Tympanoplasty type-I (myringoplasty)—to close the perforation and to improve the conductive hearing loss in large perforation.
4. Tympanoplasty plus ossiculoplasty.
5. Epidermal growth factor.

Q.18 What is tympanoplasty?

Ans. A procedure to eradicate the disease in the middle ear and to plastic reconstruct the damaged middle ear conductive mechanism with or without TM grafting.

Q.19 What are basic prerequisites?

Ans. To achieve the objective:

1. Control of infection.
2. Good cochlear reserve.
3. Patent Eustachian tube.
4. Mobile oval and round windows.

Q.20 What is objective of tympanoplasty?

Ans. The objective of tympanoplasty is the preservation or recreation of the disproportionate conductivity of the two fenestrae.

Q.21 What are the indications of tympanoplasty?

Ans. 1. Benign perforation.
  2. Dry perforation (free from infection).
  3. After the age of 8–10 years (sufficient resistance to URI).
  4. Children with both ear perforation—with conductive deafness—operated earlier.
  5. Occupation—requiring intact TM, e.g. military service.
  6. Who wish to bear hearing aid with CSOM.

Q.22 What are the contraindications of tympanoplasty?

Ans. 1. Contraindications are:
  a. Poor residual cochlear function (SNHL).
  b. Malignant neoplasm of middle or external ear.
  c. Pseudomonas infections of external or middle ear in diabetes.
  2. Relative contraindications are:
  a. Acute exacerbation of CSOM.
  b. Chronic mucoid discharge with allergic rhinosinusitis.
  c. Hidden cholesteatoma.
  d. Chronic otitis externa—caused by *Pseudomonas, Aspergillus niger* or *Staphylococcus aureus.*
  e. Eustachian tube obstruction.
  f. Only hearing ear.
  g. Better hearing ear.
  h. Advanced age.
  i. Child below 10 years.
  j. Wet ear.
  k. COPD with cough.
  l. Fixed stapes.
  m. Bleeding disorder.
  n. Septic foci in the nose, sinuses, naso or oropharynx.

Q.23 What are the basic steps of tympanoplasty?

Ans. These are:
  1. Incision—postaural or endaural.
  2. Grafting material—autograft or homografts.
  3. Tympanic repair by placing the graft underlay (inlay) or overlay (onlay) or interlay.
  4. Preparing of the bed for graft—edge freshening.
  5. Ossiculoplasty—autograft or homograft or biomaterial.
  6. Mastoid—can be exposed if disease is suspected.
  7. Grafting.
  8. Pressure packing with gelatin sponges and cotton.
  9. Dressing and bandage.

Q.24 What are various graft materials used in tympanoplasty?

Ans. Various graft materials used in tympanoplasty are:

Autografts
1. Temporalis fascia.
2. Perichondrium—tragal or chonchal.
3. Vein graft.

Homografts
1. Lyophilized dura.
2. Perichondrium.
3. Tympanic membrane.

Q.25 What are the types of myringoplasty depending on the graft placement technique?

Ans. 1. Overlay technique—graft is inserted between the outer and middle layers of the eardrum.
2. Underlay technique—the graft is inserted medial to the inner layer of the tympanic membrane.

Q.26 Why temporalis fascia is most commonly used in tympanoplasty?

Ans. Several reasons are:
1. Low BMR.
2. Thickness is almost equal to TM.
3. Easily can be obtained in plenty.
4. Can be obtained in same operative field.

Q.27 Why the underlay procedure is preferred by most of the surgeons?

Ans. 1. No epithelial cells are left under the graft so no chance of graft cholesteatoma.
2. No lateralization of graft after healing.
3. No blunting at anterior tympanomeatal angle.
4. Faster procedure.
5. Better access to middle ear.
6. Ossicular chain continuity can be assessed better.

Q.28 What are the complications of the tympanoplasty?

Ans. 1. Immediate:
    a. Bleeding.
    b. Damage of inner ear (vertigo—injury to labyrinth or labyrinthine fistulae by disease.)
    c. Facial nerve injury.
    d. Injury to dura—CSF leak.
    e. Sigmoid sinus or jugular bulb injury.
    f. Complications of anesthesia.
    g. Chorda tympani nerve injury (by stretching, drying, dissecting instruments).
2. Delayed:
    a. Infection—acute perichondritis.
    b. SNHL (damage to labyrinth, injury to stapes, labyrinth fistulae).

    c. Delayed onset of facial palsy.

    d. Failure of the graft.

    e. Conductive deafness persist.

    f. Recurrent cholesteatoma.

    g. Blunting of anterior tympanomeatal angle.

    h. Prosthesis displacement or extrusion.

Q.29 What are the types of tympanoplasty?

Ans. 1. Type I only TM is repaired.

    2. Type II ossicle maleus or incus is repaired with TM.

    3. Type III graft is placed on stapes head (Collumella effect)

    4. Type IV suprastructures of stapes are absent (Baffle effect).

    5. Type V fenestration.

    6. Type VI sono-inversion.

Q:30 What is an audiogram?

Ans. It is a graphic representation of auditory threshold responses which are obtained by testing hearing of the patient with pure tone stimuli.

Q:31 What are parameters of audiogramX?

Ans. 1. Frequency, as measured in cycles per second (Hz)

    2. Intensity as measured in decibel (db)

    The pure tone audiomety is done by measuring hearing thresholds for single frequency sounds at 250, 500, 1000, 2000, 4000, and 8000 Hz.

Q:32 What are commonly used audiogram symbols?

Ans. For left ear—X=unmasked air conduction, n=masked air conduction, >=unmasked bone conduction,]=masked bone conduction, ↓ = no response

For right ear—0=unmasked air conduction, Δ=masked air conduction, <=unmasked bone conduction, [=masked bone conduction, ↓=no response

Q:33 How wide frequency range a normal man can hear?

Ans. It is from 20 to 20,000 Hz (Adult can hear only 20–10000 Hz)

Q:34 What is speech frequency range?

Ans. It ranges from 400 to 3,000 Hz.

Q.35 What is frequency?

Ans. In short and simple, is a physical property of the sound vibration in cycle per second.

Q.36 What is pitch?

Ans. Same as of frequency but is physiological properties of sound related to speech

Q.37 What is intensity?

Ans. It is physical property of sound which is in decibels sound pressure level.

Q.38 What is loudness?

Ans. It is physiological property and is equal to intensity and is related to hearing and measured in db.

Q.39 What is decibal?

Ans. 1. It is one tenth of a bell, unit of sound. It is arbitrary unit of measurement that is logarithmic in nature. Several decibel scales are used to measure sounds and hearing.
   2. Hearing is measured in a biologic scale in decibles hearing level (dbhl).
   3. Environment sounds are measured on physical scale in decibles sound pressure level (dbspl).

Q.40 What is normal hearing level?

Ans. It is a biologic range between 10 and 20 dbhl of threshold in normal adult.

Q.41 What is hearing threshold?

Ans. It is the point at which the patient perceives a sound stimulus 50% of time.

Q.42 What is degree or grade of hearing loss?

Ans. Degree or grade of hearing level are:
   1. Nomal hearing—less than 20 db htl
   2. Mild hearing loss—20–40 db htl
   3. Moderate hearing loss—40–60 db htl
   4. Severe hearing loss—60–80 db htl
   5. Profound hearing loss—more than 80 db htl

Q.43 What is pure tone?

Ans. One single frequency to be tested.

Q.44 What is overtone?

Ans. Mixture of different frequencies.

Q.45 What is pure tone average?

Ans. It is an estimate of patients ability to hear within the speech frequencies, i.e. at 500, 1000 and 2000 Hz.

Q.46 What is masking?

Ans. Sound to the test ear can travel and perceived by the opposite ear by bone conduction through the head (transcranial transmission). This transcranial transmission is eliminated from test by masking. Masking is presentation of sound to nontest ear to prevent the nontest ear from interfering with test sound perception in the test ear.

Q.47 What difference of db of AC and BC is required for transcranial transmission?

   1. 50 db difference between the air conduction threshold between the two ears.
   2. Bone conduction sounds may crossover even at difference of 0–5 db between the two ears.

Q.48 What is air–bone gap?

Ans. It is the difference in decibels between the hearing threshold level for air and bone conduction. With normal hearing AC and BC gap is less than 15 db htl equal. In conduction HL it is significant, in SNHL it is equal but overall show a deficit

Q.49 What is head shadow effect?

Ans. When sound comes from one direction, the ear to the sound hears better than the opposite ear. The difference in hearing, threshold between two ears remain in 20 db in that situation. This is called head shadow effect.

Q.50 What is tympanometry?

Ans. It is a objective test that measures the mobility or compliance of TM and middle ear system at different pressures on either side of TM. Tympanogram—graphic representation of tympanometric results by air pressure and compliance. The compliance of TM is at maximum when air pressurs is equal to patients middle ear pressure. The range of middle ear pressure is between 0 and –150 mm of water and represents normal eustachian tube function. Middle ear pressure that is more negative than –150 are indicative of poor Eustachian tube pressure.

Q.51 What are various types of tympanograms?

Ans. 1. Type A—normal middle ear pressure
2. Type As—TM is stiffer than normal (lower compliance) with normal middle ear pressur, e.g. otosclerosis
3. Type Ad—TM is more flaccid than normal (higher compliance) with normal middle ear pressure, e.g. ossicular chain discontinuity
4. Type B—TM is not mobile, no pressure peak (middle ear effusion or perforated TM)
5. Type C—A peak in negative pressure range ($\leq$ 150 mm water), e.g. poor Eustachian tube function.

Q.52 What is ear canal physical volume test?

Ans. It is done by impedance audiometry test which measure the volume that is medial to a permatically sealed probe. It is absolute volume of ear canal in cm^3 with normal TM. The volume increases when there is perforation in TM due to additional volume of middle ear.

Q.53 What is ultrasound?

Ans. The frequencies higher than human audible range.

Q.54 What is impedance audiometry?

Ans. It consists of:
1. Tympanometry
2. Ear canal physical volume test
3. Stapedial or acoustic reflex measurement.

Q.55 What is stapedial reflex?

Ans. Stapedial muscle contracts reflexively at the onset of loud sound. Both the muscle contracts even on sound stimulation of one ear. The acoustic reflex causes immediate stiffening of ossicles and the middle ear system and TM. This can be tested by impedance or immetance audiometry.

Q.56 What is acoustic reflex neural pathways?

Ans. The acoustic reflex has both an ipsilateral and contralateral pathways. The majority of neurons passes through ipsilateral pathways:

1. Ipsilatral pathways begins at cochlea and proceeds through the nerve, cochlear nucleus, trapezoid bodies, superior olivary complex, and fascial motor nucleus to ipsilateral stapedial muscle.
2. Contralateral pathway crosses the brain stem to continue to opposite cochlear nucleus, trapezoid body, contalateral olivary complex, motor nucleaus of the fascial nerve and opposite stapedius muscle.

Q.57 What are the uses of acoustic reflex?

Ans. Measurement of acoustic reflex is valuable screening test:

1. To determine the integrity of neural pathways.
2. To detect 8th nerve tumors.
3. Cochlear hearing loss.
4. loudness tolerance test (recruitment).
5. Functional deafness.

Q.58 What is BERA?

Ans. Brainstem evoked response audiometry (BERA) is an objective, physiology measurement of hearing. It is a computerized audiometric test, used in the following:

1. Identification of retrocochlear pathology.
2. In detection of lesions which interfere with main neural hearing pathway.
3. Useful for testing hearing in infants and young childrens.
4. Used to determine hearing thresholds.

Q.59 How does BERA works?

Ans. An audiometry brainstem response is produced by sound, stimulus is perceived. A series of small electrical events (potentials) along the entire peripheral and central auditory pathways is elicited by a stimulation of ear by acoustic signals. This electrical activity is displaced as a waveform with five latency-specific wave peaks.

The latency of each wave peak corresponds to sites in the neural auditory pathways, i.e each peak represent one anatomical structure in neural pathways:

1. Wave 1—Eight nerve action potential (eight nerve nucleus situated lateral to inferior colliculus).
2. Wave II—cochlear nucleus.
3. Wave III—superior olivary complex.
4. Wave IV—lateral lemniscus.
5. Wave V—inferior colliculus.

Q.60 What is the interpretation of BERA?

Ans. 1. A tumor will slow the neural circuit and delay the waveform at the site of lesion.

2. It is used to determine the hearing thresholds by decreasing the amplitude of stimulus click, the peaks of waveform will eventually disappear.

Q.61 What is speech reception threshold (SRT)?

Ans. Speech reception threshold is the lowest intensity at which the patient correctly identifies the 50% of spoken spondee words.

Q.62 What are spondee words?

Ans. Spondee words are bisyllables compound words that are pronounced with equal emphasis on each syllable, e.g. oat-meal, popcorn, etc. these words are presented to the patient at decreasing intensities.

Q.63 What is use of SRT?

Ans. It is used to confirm the pure-tone threshold findings. The SRT should be wihin ± 6 dbs of frequencies pure-tone average.

Q.64 What is speech discrimination test?

Ans. It is used to descriminate the words to assess the understanding of speech in person.

A standerdised list (phonetically balanced list) of single syllable words are presented 30–40 db above the SRT. The score is determined according to the percentage words correctly identified by the person. A score of more than 90% is considered to represent normal word recognition and speech understanding.

Q.65 What are uses of SD?

Ans. It is used in detecting dynamic range, useful in prescribing hearing aid.

Q.66 What is phonate regression?

Ans. It is the disproportion between the pure-tone audiometry finding and speech audiometry. Pure-tone audiometry may show normal or mild degree of hearing loss while the speech discrimination is high. It is usually present in retrocochlear lesions.

Chronic Suppurative Otitis Media with Atticoantral Disease

CASE: A 35-year-old man presents with history of right ear discharge and hearing loss for last 8 years. The details of history reveals that ear discharge was incidious in onset, scanty, thick, purulent and fowl smelling and occasionally blood stained. The discharge is continous for last 8 years and mild remmision occurs only by taking some drugs and ear drops. It was not related with cold. Patient noticed diminished hearing since almost same duration with the right ear, which was incidious in onset, gradually progressive and sufficient to be noticed.

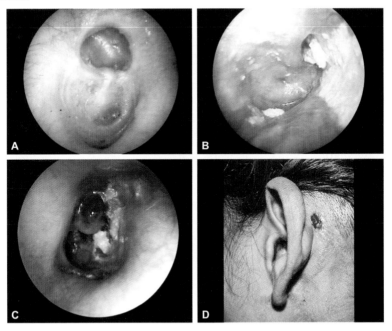

Figs 1A to D: (A) Attic extensive retraction pocket; (B) Attic disease with cholesteatoma; (C) Atticoantral disease with granulation tissue and cholesteatoma; (D) Postauricular fistula

There was not history of tinnitus, no history of giddiness and ear ache.

There is no history of any systemic disease, e.g. diabetes, hypertension, coronary artery disease, liver or kidney disease and bleeding disorders.

Similarly there was no complaints in relation to nose and throat.

Past history: Patient reveals that he tooks treatmental several occasions in his village dispensary but there was remmision in symptoms and disease did not subside completely. He has no history of any operation on the ear or any other, he has no known drug allergy.

Personal history: Patient is wood worker by profession and used to work about 8–10 hours a day with exposure to noisy atmosphere during the work. He is not habitual to smoking, chewing pan or tobacco. He is not addicted to alcohol. Food habits are normal and does not exercise but his work is associated with loss of significant calories.

Family history: He does not have any history of otosclerosis or any other disease having hearing loss or autoimmune disorder among any family member. Similarly there is no history of close contact with any family friend circle having disease like tuberculosis, syphilis, etc.

General examination: As the patient is of average built, well nourished, with no evidence of anemia or cynosis, no jaundice, no generalized lymphadenopathy, no edema feet.

Pulse: 74 per minute, BP is 120/80 mm of Hg. Respiratory rate is 16 per minute and normal, temperature is not raised.

On systemic examination: Heart and lungs are clinically normal, liver and spleen are not palpable and normal.

Examination of nose reveals no abnormality on inspection as well as no palpation.

External nose normal, nasal airway clear. On anterior rhinoscopy nasal vestibule, nasal septum; lateral wall, turbinate and meatus are normal, posterior rhinoscopy was also normal.

Examination of the oral cavity; pharynx and larynx is normal including laryngeal mirror examination.

Ear examination: In detail on inspection as well as palpation (or on probe examination) is as follows:

	Part examined	Right	Left
1.	Pinna	Normal	Normal
2.	Surrounding area		
	A Pre- and peri-auricular	NAD	NAD
	B Postauricular	Normal	
	i. Inspection	No mastoid	Normal
	ii Palpation	tenderness	No mastoid tenderness
3.	External auditory canal		
	a. Without speculum	Meatus size, wall: normal, no wax, no, discharge	Meatus size, wall: normal no wax, no discharge

Part examined	Right	Left
b. With speculum	No polyp No granulation No sagging of posteriosuperior wall	NAD
4. Tympanic membrane a. Color b. Appearance	Dull, lusterless, retracted TM adhesions, posterior-superior granulations and debris of white flakes	Pearly white Semitransparent, obliquly placed with normal visible land marks
c. Surface	Posterior-superior marginal perforation of small size with granulation and at places keratin debris, i.e. cholesteatoma	Surface is normal, no evidence of any lesion with normal cone of light present
5. Mobility	Some part is hypermobile while rest of part is tense restricted mobility	Mobility normal
6. Middle ear mucosa	Not is seen, head of stapes foot plate is seen through semitransparent TM	Not visible
7. Examination of Mastoid	No swelling, scar or fistula, retro- auricular groove— normal mastoid surface is normal and mild irregular, no tenderness	Normal
8. Eustachian tube	No opening is visible	No preparation
9. Facial nerve examination	Normal	Normal
10. Signs of CNS pathology	Nil	Nil
11. Siegl's speculum examination	Hypermobility at places retracted TM	Normal

Provisional Diagnosis: Functional Examination of Ear

Auditory functions assessed as follows:
1. Voice test; tuning fork tests:
   a. Rinnes test   BC>AC   AC>B
   b. Weber test   Laterised   Normal
                 in right ear
   c. ABC   Reduced
2. Vestibular functions—assessed by observing
   a. Spontaneous nystamus—absent
   b. Fistula test—negative on both side
   c. Positional test—not done
3. Facial nerve function tests:
   a. Taste
   b. Salivary flow test
   c. Lacrimation (Schirmer's test)

Investigations (Ears)
1. Eustachian tube function tests.
2. Radiological investigations:
   i. Xray mastoids (Law's view)
   ii. Xray chest PA view
   iii. CT scan (only in suspected complicated cases)
   iv. MRI (not required in all cases).
3. Audiological: Pure tone audiometry.
4. Swab for culture and sensitivity.
5. Seventh nerve function tests.
6. Routine hematological and urinary:
   i. Routine HB, TDLC, BT, CT
   ii. Blood for sugar, urea, creatinine
   iii. HIV
   iv. Blood chemistry
   v. Urine for complete.

Q.1 What are the main complaints of the patient?
Ans. Ear discharge and hearing loss, earache, autophony, tinnitus, itching, giddiness, headache, phonophobia (hyperacusis), diplacusis.

Q.2 What is the difference between term deafness and hearing loss?
Ans. The term deafness usually means total hearing loss to a patient. The term hearing loss is used for partial reduction in hearing capacity.

Q.3 How will you classify hearing loss ?
Ans. Hearing loss is classified into:
1. Concudctive
2. Sensorineural
3. Mixed

Conductive hearing losss—is result of impairment in sound conducting mechanism. Causes may be in the:

1. External audiotary canal—atresia, furuncle, wax, infection, polyp or tumor, and foreign body.
2. In the TM perforation—traumatic or infective origin and tympanosclerosis.
3. In Eustachian tube—obstruction, edema, malfunction.
4. Middle ear—acute otitis media, CSOM, otosclerosis, ossicular chain discontinuity, adhesive otitis media secretory otitis media, tumor, etc.

Sensorineural hearing loss results from impairment in sound perception, causes may be in:

1. Cochlear (Cochlear deafness)—Meniere's disease, labyrinthitis, ototoxic drugs, senile deafness, noise deafness .
2. Cochlear nerve (Retrocochlear deafness)—acoustic tumor, cerebellopontine angle tumor, senile deafness, toxic neuropathy.

Q.4 What does blood-stained ear discharge indicate?

Ans. It indicates presence of polyp or granulation tissue. It is also presents in carcinoma of middle ear, glomus tumor.

Q.5 What is significance of different types of ear discharage?

Ans. 1. Ear discharge is evaluated in term of quantity, color, nature and smell.
2. Discharge may be watery, mucopurulent, purulent or serosanguinous.
3. In tubotympanic disease of CSOM: Ear discharge is profuse mucopurulent or purulent (infection) or creamy or bluish nonoffencive.
4. In atticoantral disease, i.e. cholesteatoma. Ear discharge is scanty, offensive with epithelial debris and green in color (*Pseudomonas*)
5. Clear watery profuse discharge after head injury indicates CSF otorrhea.

Q.6 What is importance of tinnitus?

Ans. Tinnitus (Latin—tinnire to ring, tinkle) means ringing without any obvious external stimulus. It can ocur in any disease of the ear.

Q.7 What is significance of giddiness in CSOM ?

Ans. Giddiness (vertigo) is subjective sense of imbalance. Its occurrence in CSOM indicates intracranial complication, e.g. cerebeller abscess or labyrinthitis, it can be drug induced or independent of etiology.

Q.8 What are menings of term autophony, hyperacusis, diplacusis?

Ans: 1. Autophony—the patient hears his own voice or breath sound in his ear. It occurs in secretary otitis media and a patulous eustachian tube.
2. Hyperacusis (phonophobia)—a feeling of sense of discomfort or pain on exposure to loud sound. This usually occurs in paralysis of stapedius muscles in facial nerve palsy.
3. Diplacusis—the same tone is heard as notes of different pitch in either ear. It occurs in Meniere's disease or after stapedectomy.

Q.9 What are normal landmarks of tympanic membrane ?
Ans. 1. Handle of malleus—most important in right ear, it is at 1 o'clock position and in the left ear, it lies at 11 o'clock position.
2. The Umbo—the inferior end of the handle of malleus is situated at 'Umbo'. The cone of light (the reflection of examination light) is present from this point to anterioinferior part of TM.
3. Anterior and posterior malleolar folds separate the pars flaccida from pars tensa.
4. Cone of light.

Q.10 What are uses and advantages of the Siegle's pneumatic speculum?
Ans. 1. It is used to test the mobility of TM.
2. It gives two times magnigfication. The lens is oblique so as to be parallel to TM.
3. It is used to differentiate a thin scar from a perforation.
4. Medication—it is used to insufflate medication in the middle ear.
5. Middle ear-inner ear fistula—it is uses to elicit fistula.
6. Middle ear evacuation—it is used to clear the secretion or discharge from the middle ear.
7. It can be demonstrate as a very small or pin hole perforation.
8. It used to perform Gelle's test (Tuning fork test)
9. It is used to elicite Brown's test in glomus tumor (Blinching and pulsation sign).
10. It is used to differentitate head of malleus fixation from otosclerosis. In otosclerosis handle of malleus readily moves when applying air pressure to external canal, whereas these moments cannot be detected in fixation of head of malleus.

Q.11 How the Eustachian tube patency is tested clinically?
Ans. 1. Valsalva maneuver in adults.
2. By inflating special balloons through nose in children.
3. Toynbee maneuver.
4. Politzerization.
5. Eustachian tube catheterization.

Q12. Why does you examine the external auditory canal without ear speculum prior to with speculum?
Ans. First the ear canal is examined without ear speculum by pulling the pinna upwards and backword while the tragus is pulled forwards to spread open the meatus.
It is examined to note the:
1. Size of meatus
2. Contents of lumen
3. Swelling of its wall.
Size of meatus is essential to know for the reflection of proper size of the ear speculum to be introduced.

Q.13 How is the external canal examined with ear speculum?

Ans. Ear speculum is skeletal according to canal size. The optimum size speculun is inserted in the cartilagenous part of external auditory canal. Then canal and tympanic membrane is examined thoroughly.

Q.14 What are signs of retracted TM?

Ans. Signs of retracted TM are:
1. Apparently shortening of handle of malleus.
2. Prominence of anterior and posterior malleolar folds.
3. Prominent short process of malleus.
4. Lustreless and dull TM.
5. Distortion or displacement or absent cone of light.
6. Impaired mobility of TM.

Q.15 How is the mastoid tenderness elicited ?

Ans. Tenderness of mastoid is seen in mastoiditis and is elicited by three finger test.
1. One on the antrum (Just above and behind the meatus)
2. Over the tip.
3. Over the part between mastoid tip and mastoid antrum.

Q.16 What is our clinical diagnosis?

Ans. Chronic suppurative otitis media with atticoantral disease, i.e. postero-superior lesion granulation with cholesteatoma right ear and with conductive hearing loss.

Q.17 What is CSOM?

Ans. Chronic suppurative otitis media is a long standing infection of mucous lining of the part or whole of the middle ear cleft characterized by ear discharge and permanent perforation with variable degree of conductive deafness.

Q.18 What are types of CSOM?

Ans. 1. Tubotympanic disease (Safe or benign type): It is a long-standing infection involving mostly anterorinferior part of middle ear cleft which usually has no risk of serious complication.
2. Atticoantral disease (Unsafe as dangerous type): It is a long-standing infection involving posterosuperior part of the middle ear cleft (i.e. attic, posterosuperior part of middle ear, mastoid antrum and mastoid air cells).

The disease is often associated with high risk of serious complications.

Q.19 What is difference between atticoantral disease with tubotympanic type of CSOM?

	Tubotympanic type	Atticoantral type
1. Discharge	Profuse, mucoid, odorless	Scanty, purulent, offensive, odor
2. Perforation	Central	Attic or marginal

3. Granulations	Uncommon	Common
4. Polyp	Pale	Red and fleshy
5. Cholesteatoma	Absent	Present
6. Complications	Rare	Common
7. Deafness	Mild-to-moderate conductive	Conductive or mixed deafness

Q.20 How does atticoantral disease of CSOM manifest?

Ans. The pathological features are:
1. Cholesteatoma formation.
2. Granulation tissue with osteitis.
3. Cholestrol granuloma

It manifested in form of:
1. Attic or marginal peforation often with granulation or polyp
2. Profound conductive deafness
3. Long-standing scanty and offensive otorrhea.

Q.21 What is granulation tissue?

Ans. In short it is a tissue consisting of budding capillaries and proliferating fibroblasts. It is biological tissue response to a stimulus manifests in the form of budding newly formed capillaries and proliferating fibroblasts with variable numbers of leukocytes. The type of leukocytes infiltration depends on type of infection. In acute-polymorph, in chronic the cells are lymphocytes and in allergy mainly eosinophils. Further in unhealthy granulation tissue disinigrated WBC (pus cells) are found abundantly where as in healthy granulation the cells are healthy and scanty in number due to healing process.

Q.22 What is bacteriology of atticoantral disease?

Ans. Bacteria which causes skin infection has tendency to infect are *Pseudomonas auruginosa, B. pyocyaneus, B. proteus, E. coli.* The whole anaerobes include, *Bacteroides fragilis* and anaerobic streptococci.

Q.23 What is cholesteatoma?

Ans. The term coined by a german physiologist, Johanes Muller in 1838, who identified "a layered pearly tumor of fat". The term is misnomer because it is neither a tumor nor does it necessarily contains cholesterol crystals. Various terms subsequently used are cholesteatosis (Young), pearly tumor (Vircow), epidermosis (Tumortin), kertosis (Mc Guckin), keratoma (Schukneet). In simplest way it is "skin in the wrong place".
1. Cholesteatoma means presence of keratinizing stratified squamous epithelium within the middle ear cleft.
2. Cholesteatoma is a sac (cyst or cyst with one end opened) of keratinized squmous epithelium (matrix) resting on fibrous tissue layer.
3. Perimatrix—containing sheets of desquanted epithelial debris (keratin arranged in a concentenic layers like onion, skin like) trapped within middle ear cleft.

Thus it consists of three parts:
a. Perimatrix—outermost fibrous tissue layer.
b. Matrix (sac wall)—layer of keratized squamous epithelium.
c. Keratin debris—a central white mass comprising of sheets of desquamated epithelium produced by the matrix, arranged in concentric layers like onion skin.

Q.24 What are types of cholesteatoma?
Ans. It can be classified into:
1. Congenital
2. Acquired: (A) Primary and (B) Secondary

Q.25 What is congenital cholesteatoma?
Ans. It is an epidermal inclusion cyst arising from aberrant, embryonic, epithelial cells rests in the middle ear or mastoid behind the intact tympanic membrance without a history of ear infection.
It can be:
1. Within the TM.
2. Middle ear cleft:
   (a) Tympanic, (b) Mastoid, (c) Petrous
3. Both.
Early intratympanic pearls progress if untreated with resultant local destruction of bone and resulting disruption of TM.
Congenital cholesteatoma of the temporal bone can be found.
1. Intradural—at cerebropontine angle.
2. Extradural—in middle ear or mastoid.
It accounts for 2–5% of all cholesteatoma The incidence of middle ear congenital cholesteatoma is 1–5 % of all cholesteatoma.

Q.26 What is common presentation and growth of congenital cholesteatoma?
Ans. 1. It presents as retrotympanic middle ear mass.
2. The most common location of congenital cholesteatoma is the anterosuperior quadrant followed by posterosuperior quadrant, lesions discovered at later age are more commonly located at posterior mesotympanum.
3. Posterior located lesion affect ossicles so hearing loss is due to ossicular movement impairment or discontinuity. Anterior lesion compromises the function of Eustachian tube and causes conductive hearing loss through middle ear effusion.
4. If cholesteatoma extends to invades the labyrinth, patient may have vertigo or sensorineural deafness. Facial nerve paralysis is rare.

Q.27 What are various type of classification of congenital cholesteatoma?
Ans. 1. Derlacki and Clemis classification—lesions are classified into:
   i. Petrous pyramid
   ii. Mastoid
   iii. Tympanic.

2. Potsic classification:
    i. Stage I: Single quadrant with no ossicular or mastoid involvement (40%).
    ii. Stage II: Multiple quadrants with no ossicular or mastoid involvement (14%).
    iii. Stage III: Ossicular involvements but no mastoid involvement (23%)
    iv. Stage IV: Mastoid extension (23%)
3. Nelsons classification (Three categories):
    i. Type I: Mesotympanum with no incus or stapes erosion (15%).
    ii. Type II: Mesotympanum or attic with ossicular erosion but no mastoid extension (59%).
    iii. Type III: Mesotympanum with mastoid extension (26%).

Q.28 What is purpose of staging system of congenital cholesteatoma?
Ans. Purpose of staging system are:
1. Helpful in preoperative planning at the treatment.
2. Indicate prognosis.
3. Evaluate the result of treatment, reccurrence rate corelation.
4. Facilitate exchange information between different clinicians.
5. Assessment of manifestation and spread.

Q.29 What is pathophysiology of congenital cholesteatoma ?
Ans. The causes of congenital cholesteatoma is controversial .The various theories of pathogenesis:
1. Epithelial cell rest (Teed-Michales): Most accepted theory.
2. Invagination: Migration of squamous epithelium from deep canal wall through tympanic ring into the middle ear at weak point especially posterosuperior region.
3. Implantation (Friedberg and Sheeny): Congenital cholesteatoma is a result of implantation of squamous epithelium in to middle ear either from trauma or an unrecognized and subsequently healed tympanic membrane perforation. Reudi—ectoderm of external auditory canal may penetrate the TM in utero and migrate into middle ear.
4. Metaplasia (sade): Squamous metaplasia of the inflamed middle ear epithelium.
5. Acquired inclusion theory (TOS).

Q.30 What are findings of congenital cholesteatoma in CT scan?
Ans. 1. Computed tomography (CT) is first choice among radiologists because of its superior bony definition. It can confirm the location of middle ear mass, can determine the size of lesion.
2. Congenital cholesteatoma is usually seen as hyperdense expansile lesion, round oval in shape with well-defined margins. Lack of enhancement helps differentiating it from other lesions like neuromas, glomus tumor, sarcomas or meningioma, adenomas, metastasis.

Q.31 What are causes of white visible mass medial to TM (Retrotympanic region)?

Ans. 1. Purulent debris.
2. Congenital cholesteatoma.
3. Acquired cholesteatoma.
4. Tympanosclerosis.
5. Middle ear mass, e.g. neuroma, adenoma, abnormal developed ossicular chain.

Q.32 What are causes of vascular mass behind intact TM?

Ans. 1. Dehiscent jugular bulb.
2. Carotid artery.
3. Glomus tumor.
4. Facial neuroma.
5. Middle ear adenoma.

Q.33 What are manifestations of petrous type of congenital cholesteatoma?

Ans. It causes slowly progressively sensorineural hearing loss and loss of caloric response and facial nerve paralysis.

Q.34 What are complications of congenital cholesteatoma?

Ans. 1. Severe acute necrotizing otitis media involving bone around the antrum and petrous pyramid leading to development of bony sequestrum surrounded by infected granulation tissue with chronic otorrhea.
2. Acute suppurative otitis media—can be complicated by development of chromic osteomyelitis of nonpneumatized area of petrous bone, osteomyelitis is less likely to develop in a well-pneumatized bone because of its much lesser amount of residual marrow containing diploic bone.

Q.35 What is treatment of congenital cholesteatoma?

Ans. Surgical: Aim at complete removal of the matrix and exterization to prevent reccurrence with optimal hearing outcome.
1. In isolated anterior mesotympanum: A standard tympanoplasty approach.
2. Posterior lesions involving ossicles: Mastoidectomy.

Q.36 What is primary acquired cholesteatoma?

Ans. Sac or a pocket in the middle ear lined by keratinized squamous epithelium and contains desquamated sheets of keratin having bone eroding property without any history of previous otitis media or a preexisting perforation. It occurs in attic or posterior part of the tympanic cavity.

Q.37 What are the various theories for genesis of primary aquired cholesteatoma ?

Ans: Various theories are as follows:
1. Invagination of TM (Wittmaack's theory/ Tumarkin theory): Retraction pocket cholesteatoma persistant negative pressure (due to Eustachian

tube obstruction) in the attic causes retraction pocket which accumulate keratin debris. Then it get secondarily infected causing expansion of keratin mass. As the pocket deepens and insinuates between mucosal folds, ligaments, it becomes nonself cleaning and again increases in size.

2. Basal cell hyperplasia (Ruedi's theory): Proliferation of the basal layer of pars flaccida induced by subclinical childhood infection which subsequently form cholesteatoma, later on breaking through pars flaccida resulting in attic perforation.

3. Squamous metaplasia (Sade theory): Keratinizing squamous cell metaplasia of normal cuboidal or pavement epithelium due to subclinical infection.

4. Sudho if and Tos theory: A combination of invagination and basal cell theories for retraction pocket formation.

Q.38 What is secondary acquired cholesteatoma ?

Ans. Development of cholesteatoma secondary to an pre-existing middle ear disease with defect in the TM. Defect can be: (a) Postinfection; (b) Post injury, e.g. resulting from penetrating or blast injury; (c) Iatrogenic, e.g. after lateral graft tympanoplasty or as a complication of ventilating tube. It is often associated with posterosuperior marginal perforation or sometimes with large perforation.

Q.39 What are the various theories for pathogenesis of secondary acquired cholesteatoma?

Ans. 1. Hobermann's theory: Migration of keratinizing epithelium of external auditary canal or outer surface of TM through the perforation (involving tympanic annulus, e.g. in acute necrotizing otitis externa) in to the middle ear.

2. Metaplasia: Metaplasia of middle ear mucosa to repeated infection through preexisting perforation.

3. Implantation of viable keratinocytes into middle ear cleft through marginal perforation.

Q.40 What are the various types of acquired cholesteatoma of the middle ear?

Ans. TOS proposed the classification as follows:

1. Attic cholesteatoma: It arises from shrapnel's membrane and extends primarily into attic.

2. Sinus cholesteatoma: It arises at posterosuperior retraction of pars tensa and extends primarily into tympanic sinus. Then it spreads to the incus body into posterior attic and antrum.

3. Tensa retraction cholesteatoma: Arises from an entirely retracted tensa draping over the posterior and anterior wall of middle ear, extending into hypotympanum and tubal orifice, later on it may extend medially to malleus folds towards the posterior and anterior attic.

Q.41 What is importance of TOS classification of acquired cholesteatoma?

Ans. It is important for the evaluation of natural history, prognosis, surgical methods and results.

Q.42 What is mechanism of bone destruction in cholesteatoma?

Ans. 1. Pressure-induced bone resorption (ischemic necrosis).
    2. Enzymatic dissolution—by cytokine mediated inflammation by collagenase produced by perimatrix.
    3. Bone demineralization—hyperemic demineralization.
    4. Chemical theory—liberation of chemicals at perimatrix.

Q.43 Why the bacteria, secondarily infecting cholesteatoma, is resistant to antibiotics?

Ans. Otopathogenic strains of *Pseudomonas aeruoginosa* are capable of providing biofilm and become highly resistant to antimicrobial therapy. Bacterial proliferation and super infection of accumulated debris form a biofilm that leads to chronic infection and epithelial proliferation, which is enhanced by cytokine-mediated inflammatory response.

Q.44 What is effect of cholesteatoma on ossicles?

Ans. Ossicular necrosis: Commanly long process of incus, suprastructure of stapes, handle of malleus and even entire chain may be destroyed.

Q.45 How does granulation or polyp develop in atticoantral disease?

Ans. Sometimes low-grade osteitis of bone, margin of notch of Rivinus or posterosuperior meatal wall occurs. There may be granulation tissue formation. Mucoperiosteal or mucoendosteal involvement may occur due to chronic inflammation resulting in aural polyp formation.

Q.46 What is cholesterol granuloma?

Ans. It may occur as a single entity or in combination with granulations or cholesteatoma. It usually occurs at the site of capillary hemorrhage in the middle ear effusion.

Histopathology: It consists of granulation tissue with deposition of cholesterol crystals surrounded by foreign body giant cells.

Q.47 What is black cholesteatoma?

Ans. It is rare type, which is dark colored due to dark secretion and old hemorrhages.

Q.48 What is the difference between granulation and polyp?

Ans. Granulation and marginal polyp are secondary to chronic osteitis. Polyp is pedunculated and single. Granulations are multiple and sessile. They are composed of chromic inflammatory cells in a vascular connective tissue stroma.

They usually arise from:
1. Attic
2. Posterior-superior margin of TM
3. Promontory

4. Eustachian tube orifice
5. Aditus ad antrum
6. Lateral semicircular canal area
7. Fallopian canal.

Q.49 What is Prussak's space?
Ans. Prussak's space is superior recess and is behind the TM. It is bounded laterally by Sharpnell's membrance, medially by neck of the malleus and inferiorly by short process of malleus and superiarly enclosed by the lateral malleolar fold in the middle ear.

Q.50 Why is Prussak's space significant?
Ans. A retraction pocket or perforation starts at this potential space which allow to accumulate keratin debris to enter the middle ear space.

Q.51 What are causes of expansion of cholesteatoma?
Ans. 1. Moisture
2. Infection
3. Failure of mucous barrier.

Q.52 What are various symptoms of atticoantral disease of CSOM?
Ans. 1. Ear discharge—scanty, fowl smelling, purulent, as greenish (Pseudomonas infection); blood stained (granulation tissue formed) total cessation of discharge is due to seal of perforation by crust, inflammatory mucosa or a polyp; is liable to result in complication.
2. Hearing loss—conductive type of variable degree: Initially mild, gradually progress to moderate degree (due to destructive process) may be mixed if inner ear is involved. Sometimes hearing may be normal if cholesteatoma bridges the gap between TM and stapes.
3. Tinnitus—can occur.
4. Giddiness—indicates spread of infection to labyrinth.
5. Symptoms of complication like earache, giddiness with nausea and vomiting, headache, facial deformity (facial nerve paralysis), fever.

Q.53 What are signs or findings in atticoantral type of CSOM?
Ans. There can be:
1. Perforation of TM—attic perforation in Sharpnell membrane, marginal perforation in posterosuperior region.
2. Retracted TM and pocket of variable degree—invagination of TM in attic or at posteriosuperior area of pars tansa or in the posterior part of pars tansa or whole of TM in all direction.
3. Cholesteatoma—pearly white flakes of cholesteatoma present in retraction pocket.
4. Granulation—reddish in color at attic or posterosuperior region or on promontory.
5. Polyp—Red congested, pedunculated with irregular surface at posterosuperior region.
6. Sagging down of posterosuperior canal wall—due to excessive cholesteatoma within mastoid antrum.

7. Tenderness on mastoid antrum—suggests mastoid bone involvement.
8. Swelling in mastoid region—results from mastoid abscess.
9. Conductive hearing loss—of variable degree even may be mixed (degeneration of cochlear hair cells).
10. Fistula sign—may be positive.

Q.54 Why does complications occur in atticoantral disease of CSOM?
Ans. Complications occur because of:
1. Ossicles obstruct the drainage of pus.
2. Site of pathology is surrounded by many vital structures (facial nerve, semicircular canal, tegmen, lateral sinus)
3. Bone eroding nature of disease.
4. Infecting organisms are usually resistant to common antibiotics.

Q. 55 What is mastoid reservoir phenomemon?
Ans. It is characterized by profuse and persisting discharge even after best of conservative therapy and hazy mastoid air cells on X-ray. Cortical mastoidectomy is indicated in such cases even in tubotympanic type of CSOM.

Q.56 What is pathogenesis of cholesteatoma?
Ans. 1. Focal area—are pars flaccida, posterior superior part of tensa and adjacent skin of deep external auditory canal.
2. Expansion of focal area—depends on ventilatory anatomy of middle ear, Eustachian tube, pneumatization of mastoid and destruction of mucosal ligaments, folds or adhesions.
3. Eustachian tube obstruction—causes vaccum in middle ear and retraction of TM, and dimple formation.
4. Retraction pocket—dimple deepens but fundus is still visible. It occurs either at Prossak's space or posterosuperior part of pars tensa.
5. Formation of sac with enlargement.
6. Expansion of cholesteatoma into the middle ear, aditus ad antrum and mastoid antrum.
7. Destruction of bones and low grade osteitis.
8. Osteitis and granulation.
9. Stage of complications or stagnation process or healing process or natural radical mastoidectomy.

Q.57 What is masked mastoiditis?
Ans. It is characterized by:
1. Result of inadequate treatment of acute otitis media.
2. Latent infection in pneumatized mastoid.
3. Tender mastoid.
4. Conductive hearing loss.

Q.58 Which finding in X-ray is definitely suggestive of mastoiditis?
Ans. Intracellular breakdown in pneumatized mastoid.

Q.59 What are X-ray findings in atticoantral type of CSOM?
Ans. 1. Hypocellular or acellular mastoid.
2. Erosion of ossicles.
3. Cavitation.

Q.60 What are various types of mastoid abcess?
Ans. There are:
1. Subperiosteal abscess.
2. Bezold's abscess.
3. Muret's abscess.
4. Citelli's abscess.
5. Luc's abscess (Zygomaticitis).
6. Petrositis.
7. Extradural (Epidural) abscess.

Q.61 What is subperiosteal mastoid abscess?
Ans. Subperiosteal abscess—it develops at suprameatal triangle, pus from the antrum, spreads through vascular channels. In some there may be protrusion of posterosuperior meatal wall.

Q.62 What are features of Luc's abscess?
Ans. These are:
1. Pus escapes from zygomatic cells to form abscess deep to temporal muscle.
2. It produce swelling above and infront of ear (preauricular swelling)
3. Edema of upper lid.

Q.63 What is Bezold's abscess?
Ans. Bezold's abscess—results from suppuration of lateral group (external group) of mastoid tip cells and pus travels from tip of mastoid along the sternomastoid muscle and form at lateral neck.

Q.64 What is Muret's abscess?
Ans. Muret's abscess results from suppuration of medial group (inner side) of mastoid tip cells and pus travels from this area along the digastric muscle in to the digastric fossa (submandibular region). In these patients, trismus may be observed.

Q.65 What is petrous abscess?
Ans. Petrous abscess—spread of infection to petrous apex may involve the cavernous sinus and lead to paralysis of VIth nerve and pain in the trigeminal nerve (Gradinigo's syndrome).

Q.66 What is extradural abscess?
Ans. It is also called epidural abscess; pus collects between dura and bone.

Q.67 What are various tests to assess functional impairment occurring in atticoantral disease?

Ans. 1 Hearing tests:
  a. Voice test, CV and WC
  b. Tuning fork test, Rinne test, Weber test and ABC
  c. Audiometry
2. Vestibular test:
  a. Spontaneous nystagmus
  b. Fistula sign
  c. Positional nystagmus
  d. Doll eye test
3. Eustachian tube function tests:
  a. History
  b. Valsalva
  c. Toynbee
  d. Eustachian catheterization
4. Facial nerve function—may be normal, or sign of paresis/paralysis.

Q.68 What are various investigations done in CSOM?

Ans. Pneumonic EARS:
1. Eustachian tube patency.
2. Audiometry pure tone—conductive hearing loss.
3. Radiological—(a) X-ray mastoid (Law's view); (b) CT scan; (c) MRI.
4. Swab for culture and sensitivity—for selection of antibiotic for local and systemic use.

Q. 69 Why is X-ray done in CSOM?

Ans. 1. To know the pneumatization.
2. Position of dura and lateral sinus for any evidence of destruction.
3. Extension of lesion by cavity formation with sclerosed margin.

Q.70 What is natural radical mastoidectomy?

Ans. In some cases successive healing may occur by limiting of disease process and extension of cholesteatoma. Natural radical mastoidectomy may result from absorption of bone at outer attic or deep posterior medial wall with extension of cholesteatoma.

Q.71 What is false fundus?

Ans. A false fundus is a thin membrane partial or complete, present at the isthmus of external auditory canal as a result of healing process in CSOM.

Q.72 What is treatment of atticoantral type of CSOM?

Ans. Treatment depends on stages of CSOM:
  I. Active stage:
    a. With cholesteaoma—mastoid surgery
    b. With polyp—polypectomy may be tried then if needed mastoid surgery

    c. With granulation—remove or reduce granulate then followed by mastoid surgery

    d. Retraction pocket—antibiotics or suction clearance under microscope and periodic inspection.

  II. Quiscent stage: Under monthly observation for 6 months. If discharge recur treatment is modified radical matoidectomy.

  III. Inactive stage: Permanent precaution and hearing aid.

  IV. Stage of complication: Mastoid surgery.

Q.73 What is residual cholesteatoma ?

Ans. Squamous epithelium not removed from middle ear cleft in cholesteatoma surgery. Cholesteatoma can be left at over a lateral canal fistula or on a stapedial crus.

Q.74 What is recurrent cholesteatoma?

Ans. 1. A cholesteatoma that develops from the retraction pocket in to the middle ear epitympanum or facial recess or from ingrowth of skin secondary to graft failure.

    2. It usually occurs in cases operated like in intact canal wall technique (in 20% cases) or in cases where wall was reconstructed (in 5%cases).

Q.75 What are the precautions to prevent recurrent cholesteatoma?

Ans. To avoid recurrence of cholesteatoma, adhesion between lateral and medial wall must be prevented, Eustachian tube patency must be obtained in postoperative period.

CASE

13

Chronic Suppurative Otitis Media with Ear Polyp

CASE: A patients presents with history of ear discharge and loss of hearing since 6 years. On examination there is a small smooth ovoid to rounded globular mass in the external auditory canal occupying whole of the lumen of the canal. Polyp is not painful, soft in consistency and not friable and does not bleed. By pressuring the polypoidal mass, patient does not feel giddiness and no nystagmus was observed and no facial twitchings were seen.

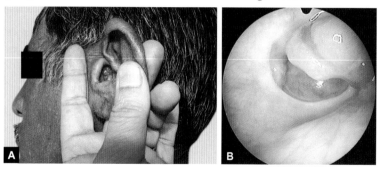

Figs 1A and B: (A) Polyp in left external auditory meatus; (B) Polyp coming out from middle ear, part of tympanic membrane is visible

Provisional Diagnosis: CSOM with Ear Polyp

Q.1 What is ear polyp?
Ans. It arises from middle ear as a prolapsed mucous membrane or as a pedunculated granuloma.

Q.2 What are points in favor of polyp?
Ans. Polyp is smooth, ovoid or rounded or globular mass, pale gray or pearly white in color, sometimes pinkish in color, lying in external auditory canal (Fig. 1A) after its origin from medial wall of middle ear. It is pedunculated, soft in consistency, nonfriable and does not bleed on touch.

Q.3 The patient feels vertigo on pressing the polyp with probe. What does this signify?
Ans. It means polyp is arising from lateral semicircular canal with underlying osteitis and fistula.

Q.4 Facial twitching is seen on pressing the polyp with probe. What does this signify?

Ans. It means the polyp is arising from fallopian (facial) canal with underlying osteitis with impending facial nerve paralysis.

Q.5 What are various lesions of the external auditory canal, which can mimic an ear polyp?

Ans. Polypoidal lesions arising in the external ears are:
1. Granuloma: Caused by unhealed furuncle or traumatic ulcer, or as a result of irritation cause by wax, keratosis obsturans, foreign body or debris.
2. Tumors: Lesions like ceruminoma, papilloma, exostosis and malignant lesion.

Q.6 What are the various lesions of the middle ear, which can mimic a ear polyp?

Ans. Polypoidal mass arising from the middle ear can be:
1. Simple polyp with tubotympanic disease of the ear (Fig. 1B).
2. Granulomatous polyp with atticoantral disease.
3. Glomus tumor.
4. Malignant neoplasm—carcinoma.

Q.7 What are the types of polyp in case of CSOM?

Ans. Two type:
1. Simple polyp: Arising from medial wall of the middle ear in tubotympanic disease without evidence of osteitis of underlying bone. It is smooth, soft and dose not bleed on touch.
2. Granulomatous polyp: It usually arises from attic or posterosuperior part of pars tensa or deep canal wall and is associated with atticoantral disease with evidence of osteitis or bone erosions. It is friable and can bleed on touch.

Q.8 What are the investigations to be done in ear polyp?

Ans. 1. Hearing examination: By tuning fork tests (Audiometry).
2. Ear swab for culture and sensitivity.
3. X-ray mastoid: Law's view.
4. CT scan: If tumor is suspected.
5. Biopsy.

Q.9 What is treatment?

Ans. 1. Polypectomy: In case of inflammatory polyp by aural snare or punch biopsy. Polyp arising from middle ear should not be avulsed to prevent ossicular disruption.
2. Mastoid surgery or tympanoplasty later on depending on type of pathology.

Q.10 What are the advantages of simple polypectomy?

Ans. Polypectomy:
1. Helps in drainage of middle ear.
2. Permits better visualization of TM for proper diagnosis and subsequent treatment.

Multiple Perforations of the Tympanic Membrane

CASE: Multiple small perforations seen in the anterior part of tympanic membrane (Figs 1A and B).

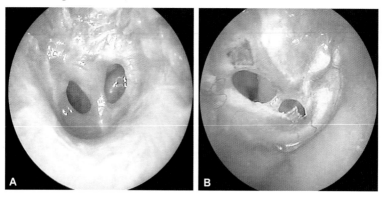

Figs 1A and B: (A) Two perforations in pers tensa; (B) Multiple perforations with congested TM and patches of myringosclerosis

Provisional Diagnosis: Tubercular Otitis Media

Q.1 What are the special features of tubercular otitis media?
Ans. 1. Multiple perforations of TM (Figs 1A and B).
  2. Painless pale granulation.
  3. Early and more frequent complication.
  4. Hearing loss is out of proportion to disease.

Q.2 What are the causes of multiple perforation of TM?
Ans. 1. Tuberculous otitis media.
  2. Traumatic blast injury specially in bomb blast.
  3. Otomycosis.
  4. Postmyringoplasty.
  5. Healed otitis media with atelectasis.
  6. Erroneous application of some chemicals, e.g. caustic or silver nitrate.

Q.3 Why does multiple perforations occur in tuberculosis?
Ans. Multiple tubercles are formed at many sites in the middle ear which coalesce and then results in multiple perforation. Later on these join to form a large subtotal perforation.

Q.4 What are the common complications of tuberculous otitis media?
Ans. Complications are:
1. Labyrinthitis
2. Tubercular meningitis
3. Facial paralysis.

Q.5 How diagnosis is confirmed?
Ans. 1. Routine histological examination of middle ear surgery during surgery.
2. Routine X-ray of chest PA view.
3. PCR for TB.

Q.6 What are the characteristic features of perforation of TM in tuberculosis?
Ans. 1. The discharge is serosanguinous or sometimes blood-stained.
2. The edge of perforation is pale, thin and undermined.
3. There is associated granulation even in central perforation.

Q.7 Name the types of tuberculosis of the middle ear.
Ans. Two types:
1. Primary tuberculosis of the ear seen in children.
2. Secondary to pulmonary tuberculosis—common in young adult with extensive sputum positive chest tuberculosis.

Q.8 What is the treatment?
Ans. Antitubercular therapy.

Bell's Palsy

CASE: A 40-year-old man presents with complaints of pain around the ear, epiphora and inability to close the right eye, deviation of mouth towards left-side for last 2 days. He gives history of exposure to cold winds 3 days back.

On examination, there was an evidence of infranuclear facial palsy with loss of forehead wrinkle, partial closure of right eye, drooping of corner of mouth, deviation of mouth to opposite side and positive Bell's phenomenon, chorda tympani nerve was found congested on otoscopy.

Provisional Diagnosis: Infranuclear Facial Paralysis—Bell's Palsy

Q.1 What is Bell's palsy?

Ans. Bell's palsy is acute unilateral paresis or paralysis of the face of unknown etiology. It is labelled as Bell's palsy only after exclusion of other causes.

Q.2 What is sex incidence of Bell's palsy?

Ans. 1. Females in teen age and twenties have a predilection.
  2. Equal sex ratio in middle age group.
  3. Slight male preponderance in older age group.

Q.3 What are the various conditions or diseases which associate or influence the Bell's palsy?

Ans. These are pregnancy, diabetes, AIDS, etc.
  1. Bell's palsy is three times more common in pregnancy.
  2. It is more common in diabetes.
  3. It is more common in AIDS patients.

Q.4 What is etiology of Bell's palsy?

Ans. 1. Viral infection: Herpes simplex virus type (HSV) is claimed to be associated with it. There is a high prevalence of HSV antibodies in these patients.
  2. Immunogenic theory: Immunogenic injury as a potential cofactor in Bell's palsy as suggested by presence of segmental demylination of nerve with lymphocytic infiltration in perineurium of nerve.

3. Ischemia: Vasospasm causes ischemia leading to edema of connective tissue in facial nerve canal and elevation of intraneural pressure producing venous stasis and stagnation of capillary flow and more compression of nerve further occurs.

Q.5 What are the sites of lesion in Bell's palsy?

Ans. 1. Meatal trauma at entrance of the labyrinthine part (commonest part)
2. At stylomastoid foramen
3. At descending part of nerve.

Q.6 What is the histopathology of Bell's palsy?

Ans. Hyperemia of the nerve sheath, oedema of nerve, wallerian degeneration with vascular engorgement.

Q.7 What is Wallerian degeneration?

Ans. The process of degeneration of an axon after injury is called Wallerian degeneration.

Q.8 What is rate of regeneration?

Ans. Rate of regeneration of an axon is 1 mm day provided neurilemmal tube is intact. Recovery occurs in 10–14 weeks.

Q.9 What is Bell's phenomenon?

Ans. On attempt to close the eye, the globe of the eyeball move upwards.

Q.10 What are the various types of nerve lesion?

Ans. The lesion may be due to compression, crushing, cutting, stretching, cold, heat, cautery or anesthesia.

Q.11 What are the various types of nerve injury?

Ans. According to Seddon's classification, the various types of nerve injury are as follows:
1. Neuropraxia: Conduction of nerve fibers is blocked at the site of lesion but distal to lesion, the nerve action potential is normal. Complete recovery occurs.
2. Axonotmesis: Axon is severed (cut) leading to wallerian degeneration distal to injury site. Recovery is associated with axonal sprouting and nerve degeneration.
3. Neurotmesis: If nerve trunk is cut or complete transection occurs, no functional recovery is anticipated.

Q.12 What are the various clinical features of Bell's palsy?

Ans. 1. History of exposure to cold wind may be present.
2. Sudden onset with unilateral involvement of face.
3. Pain around ear.
4. Features of muscle weakness:
   – Bell's phenomenon—upwards movement of eye ball on attempting to close the eye (Fig. 1A)
   – Epiphora due to loss of blinking
   – Deviation of mouth to opposite side (Fig. 1B)

        – Drooping of corner of mouth
        – Loss of wrinkle of forehead
5. Loss of taste
6. Phonophobia, hyperacusis, absent stapedial reflex
7. Chorda tympani nerve may be congested on otoscopy.

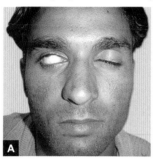 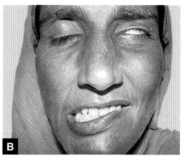

Figs 1A and B: (A) Inability to close the right eye and upward rolling of the eyeball (Bell's phenomenon); (B) Lower half left facial palsy

Q.13 What are the various investigations of diagnosis?
Ans. 1. History.
      2. Clinical examination.
      3. Complete ear examination.
      4. Topognostic tests
          – Schirmer's test for lacrimation
          – Test for taste sensation—chemical gustometry or electrogustometry
          – Test for taste for salivation—salivary flow test
          – Stapedial reflex tests.
      5. Electrodiagnostic test
          – Nerve excitability tests (NET)
          – Maximal stimulation test (MST)
          – Electroneurography (ENOG) or evoked electromyography
          – Electromyography.
      6. Radiological: CT scan and MRI.

Q.14 What is the treatment for Bell's palsy?
Ans. Treatment is supportive, medical and surgical:
      1. Supportive treatment
          – Reassurance of patient
          – Application of moist heat over the affected side
          – Facial exercise and physiotherapy
          – Eye care to prevent exposure keratitis
          – Preventive measures are artificial tears (methyl-cellulose) eye-ointment at night, adhesive tape at corner of eye during sleep, goggles during day time.
      2. Medical treatment
          – Vasodilator nicotinic acid can be tried
          – Antiviral therapy. Acyclovir 500 mg QID for 5 days in early stage

- Steroid prednisolone 1 mg/kg body weight in divided doses in tapering method
- Vitamin B_1, B_6 and B_{12}.
3. Surgical treatment
  - Decompression of nerve
  - Tarsorrhaphy
  - Facial nerve repair.

Q.15 What is the role of steroid in Bell's palsy?

Ans. 1. It is helpful to reduce the risk of degeneration if given in early state.
  2. To prevent or lessen synkinesis.
  3. May prevent progression to complete paralysis.
  4. To hasten recovery.
  5. To prevent autonomic synkinesis (Crocodile tears).

Q.16 What is the criteria for indication of surgical decompression?

Ans. Serial electroneurography is done every third day, from fourth day of onset of Bell's palsy till the 11th day. If during this period, the degeneration is more than 90% decompression of the facial nerve is indicated otherwise medical treatment is continued.

Q.17 What is the indication of lateral tarsorrhaphy?

Ans. It is done to prevent exposure keratitis, and its complications (Bad syndrome), these are:
  1. Bell's phenomenon absent
  2. Anesthesia of cornea
  3. Dryness of eyes.

Q.18 What is grading of facial paralysis (House and Brackmann)?

Ans. 1. Grade I: Normal
  2. Grad II (Mild dysfunction): Slight weakness on close inspection, normal symmetry at rest, moderate to good forehead function, complete eye closer is possible. Slight asymmetry of mouth.
  3. Grade III (Moderate dysfunction): Obvious difference between two sides, notable synkinesis, normal symmetry and tone at rest.
  4. Sight to moderate movement of forehead, complete closure of eye without effort, slight weak with maximal efforts.
  5. Grade IV (Moderate to severe): Obvious weak and disfiguring asymmetry. At rest normal symmetry and tone, slight to moderate movement at forehead, complete closure of eye with efforts, mouth asymmetry is affected.
  6. Grade V (Severe): Hardly perceptible motion, asymmetry at rest, no movement of forehead, incomplete eye closure, slight movement of mouth.
  7. Grade VI (Total paralysis): No movement.

Q.19 What is facial nerve?

Ans. It is seventh cranial nerve which is a mixed nerve having both motor and sensory roots.

1. Motor supplies the muscle of facial expression and some other muscles.
2. The sensory roots has three components:
   - Parasympathetic efferent fibers: Secretomotor to the lacrimal, submandibular and sublingual salivary glands and nasal mucous glands
   - Affernt fibers conveying taste sensation from the anterior two-thirds of the tongue
   - Cutaneous sensation fibers from the Ramsay Hunt area in the external auditory meatus.

Q.20 What is the course of facial nerve?
Ans. Facial nerve is 60–70 mm in length. It is divided into three parts:
   1. Intracranial part (15–20 mm)
      - Motor root
      - Sensory root
      - Pontine segment (23–24 mm)
      - Meatal segment (7–8 mm).
   2. Intratemporal part
      - Labyrnthine part (4 mm)
      - Tympanic and horizontal part (12–13 mm)
      - Mastoid or vertical part (15–20 mm).
   3. Extratemporal part
      - Extend from stylomastoid foramen to peripheral division of the facial nerve.

Q.21 What are the various branches of facial nerve in intratemporal region?
Ans. 1. Greater superficial petrosal nerve arises from the geniculate ganglion, contains secretomotar fibres to lacrimal gland and nasal mucosal glands.
   2. Lesser superficial petrosal nerve arises from the geniculate ganglion.
   3. Nerve to stapedious arises from vertical part and supplies the stapedius muscle.
   4. Chorda tympani nerve arises from vertical part, passes between the incus and malleus, carries taste sensation from anterior two-thirds of tongue and secretomotor to submandibular and sublingual salivary gland.

Q.22 What are the branches of facial nerve in parotid space?
Ans. 1. Postauricular branches arises near stylomastoid foramen supply the occipitofrontalis and postural muscles.
   2. Digastric branch arises near to stylomastoid foramen and supply the posterior belly of digastric muscle.
   3. Stylomastoid branch may arises from digastric branch to supply the stylohyoid muscle.

Q.23 What are the various terminal branches?
Ans. 1. Frontal branch.
   2. Temporal branch to intrinisic muscle.

3. Zygomatic branch to orbicularis oculi.
4. Buccal branch facial muscle.
5. Marginal mandibular branch risoris as muscle of lower lip.
6. Cervical branch to platysma.

Q.24 Explain the system of blood supply to the facial nerve?

Ans. • Blood supply of intracranial part:
  – Anterior-inferior cerebellar artery
  – Branch from internal auditory artery
• Blood supply of intratympanic part:
  – Superficial petrosal artery arise from middle meningeal artery.
  – Stylomastoid artery arise from posterior auricular artery.

These two vessel system anastomose together at the level of oval window over the facial nerve.

Q.25 What is microanatomy of the facial nerve?

Ans. Motor division of facial nerve contains almost 7000 axons. Nerve contains endoneurium and perineurium.

Q.26 What are radiological investigations to assess the facial nerve paralyses?

Ans. X-ray of the mastoids:
1. Submentovertical (Hurst View): Stylomastoid foramen.
2. Towne's view: For internal auditory canal.
3. Stenver's view: For internal auditory meatus.
4. CT scan: fallopian canal.
5. MRI: Facial nerve.

Q.27 What are the various surgical landmarks to identify facial nerve in the middle-ear and mastoid?

Ans. 1. Lateral semicircular canal: Above to the digastric ridge below lateral semicircular canal, most crucial landmark, second genu hugs the inferior aspect of the lateral semicircular canal.
2. Incus: It lies lateral to facial nerve.
3. Digastric ridge: Anterior end of the digastric ridge points to the lateral and inferior aspect of vertical part.
4. Stylomastoid foramen: Nerve exits through it.
5. Chorda tympani nerve.
6. Process cochleoriformis: It represents the site of geniculate ganglion which lies just anterior to it.
7. Oval window nicke: Facial nerve lies above oval window.
8. Blood vessels along the vertical portion and 2nd genu of facial nerve are useful guides for location of facial nerve when bleeding is increased (sentinel bleeding) during mastoid surgery, indicate closeness of nerve.
9. Cog: A spine of bone hangs inferiorly from Tegmen (anterior attic plate). Facial nerve lies anterior to cog just before it turns into 1st genu.

Q.28 What are the surgical landmarks to identify the facial nerve in the extracranial region?

Ans. 1. Trager points: Nerve is located 1 cm deep and inferior to anteromedial edge of the tragus cartilage.
2. Tympanomastoid suture: Facial nerve is 5 mm inferior to this part where it bisects the angle between the tympanic plate and the posterior belly of digastric.
3. Styloid process: Nerve course lateral to the styloid process at its base.
4. Retromandibular vein: Facial nerve passes superficial to the vein.
5. Identification of peripheral branches.

Q.29 Name the tests which help in assessing progression facial nerve paralysis?

Ans. 1. Stapedial reflex (Impedence audiometry).
2. Electroneurography.
3. Maximal stimulation.
4. Nerve excitability.

Q.30 Which tests are useful in diagnostic assessment of facial nerve?

Ans. 1. Blink reflex.
2. Electromyography.
3. Electroneurography.

Q.31 What is Melkersson Rosenthal syndrome?

Ans. It is characterized by recurrent sudden peripheral facial nerve palsy, painless swelling of lip, face and fissured tongue.

Q.32 What are the various causes of bilateral facial paralysis?

Ans. The various causes of bilateral facial paralysis are:
1. Guillain-Barre syndrome.
2. Leukemia.
3. Bulbar palsy.
4. Skull fracture.
5. Moebious syndrome.
6. Sarcoidosis.
7. Bell's palsy.

Q.33 What is Antonis palsy?

Ans. It is like Bell's palsy. It is a viral prodrone and features are facial weakness, pain, epiphora, loss of taste, hyperacusis and decreased lacrimation. Other cranial nerves V, IX and II cervical and vagus nerve may be involved.

Q.34 What is Lyme's disease?

Ans. It also called Bannwarth's syndrome. It is characterized by rash, fever, myalgia, arthralgia, pharyngitis, lymphadenopathy, facial nerve palsy (unilateral or bilateral)

Q.35 What are various sequelae of facial nerve palsy?

Ans. 1. Facial ticks.
2. Synkinesis.

3. Crocodile tear.
4. Frey's syndrome.
5. Gustatory rhinorrhea syndrome.
6. Gustatory otorrhea syndrome.

Q.36 What is crocodile tears?

Ans. Lacrimation during eating, due to misdirection of secretomotor, impulses for salivary glands and treated by tympanic neurectomy.

Q.37 Why is facial nerve paralysis according to degree of severity?

Ans. According to Sunderland classification:
    I.   Degree: Compression
    II. Degree: Interruption of axoplasm and myelin
    III. Degree: Disruption at endoneurium
    IV. Degree: Disruption of endoneurium and perineurium
    V.   Degree: Transection of nerve

Q.38 Why is the function of forehead muscles, preserved in supranuclear lesion?

Ans. Motor nucleus of facial nerve in the pons receive fibers from both cerebral hemisphere which innervates forehead muscles. Therefore, the function of forehead muscle is preserved in supranuclear lesion, but not in infranuclear lesion.

Q.39 Why is the emotional movements such as smiling and crying is preserved in supranuclear facial palsies?

Ans. Facial nucleus receive fibres from the thalamus by alternate route which is responsible for involuntary control of facial muscles. Therefore, emotional movement like smiling and crying are preserved in supranuclear palsies.

Q.40 What are the various passive signs for muscle test in facial nerve palsy?

Ans. Passive signs are asymmetry of:
    1. Palpebral border.
    2. Nasolabial fold.
    3. Vermillian border.

Q.41 What are the various active signs for testing the affected muscles in facial nerve palsy?

Ans. 1. Frontalis—frowning the forehead.
    2. Orbicularis oculi—close the eye.
    3. Buccinator—blowing the check.
    4. Orbicularis oris—movement of angle of mouth.
    5. Platysma—neck muscle contraction when patient drows the angle of mouth while stiffening the neck muscle.

Q.42 What are the various muscles which could not be tested clinically in facial nerve paralysis?

Ans. 1. Posterior belly of digastric muscle.
    2. Stylohyoid.

3. Occipital belly of occipitofrontalis.
4. Muscles of pinna.

Q.43 What are the causes of facial paralysis?

Ans. Causes of facial nerve paralysis are classified as follows:
1. Intracranial causes.
2. Intratemporal causes.
3. Extratemporal causes.
4. General or systemic causes.

Q.44 What are the various intracranial causes of facial nerve paralysis?

Ans. Intracranial causes are as follows:
1. In the brainstem:
   - Vascular: Thrombosis, embolism, hemorrhage
   - Trauma: To brainstem, head injury
   - Infection: Polio, diphtheria, infective neuritis, brain abscess
   - Tumors: Pontine ganglioma.
2. Between brainstem and internal auditory canal (cerebropontine angle):
   - Trauma: Fracture of base of skull, surgery of V nerve and VIIIth nerve
   - Meningitis: Nonspecific, tuberculosis, syphilis
   - Tumours: Acoustic neuroma, CP angle tumor
   - Metastatic carcinoma
   - Congenital cholesteatoma.

Q.45 What are intratemporal causes of facial palsy?

Ans. Ninety percent of cases at infranuclear facial palsy are due to intratemporal causes. Bell's palsy accounts for 66% of such cases.

Intratemporal causes are as follows:
1. Idiopathic: Bells palsy, Melkersson's syndrome.
2. Trauma:
   - Surgical—in mastoid surgery, tympanoplasty and stapedectomy
   - Accidental—fracture of temporal bones, contusional injury, penetrating injury.
3. Infection:
   - Bacterial—acute supportive otitis media, chronic suppurative otitis media, tuberculous otitis media, malignant otitis externa
   - Virus—herpes zoster otitis, Antoni's palsy.
4. Tumors:
   - Benign tumor—glomus tumor
   - Malignant primary—carcinoma of external or middle ear and sarcomatous tumor
   - Metastatic tumor of temporal bone
   - Facial nerve tumors.

Q.46 What are the extratemporal causes of facial palsy?

Ans. The extratemporal causes are:
1. Trauma
    - Birth trauma (forceps delivery and difficult labor)
    - Surgical—parotid surgery
    - Accidental injury
2. Tumor: Parotid malignancy and metastasis in parotid lymph nodes.

Q.47 What are the various systemic diseases which can cause facial nerve paralysis?

Ans. The various systemic diseases are:
1. Congenital agenesis: Very rare.
2. Diabetes, hypothyroidism.
3. Lead poisoning.
4. Infection: Polio, diphtheria, syphilis, leprosy, sarcoidosis.
5. Leukemia.
6. Acute porphyria.
7. Wegener's granulomatosis.
8. Uremia.
9. Polyarteritis nodosa.
10. Demyelinating disease.

Q.48 What is the difference between supranuclear and intranuclear facial nerve palsy?

Ans. The difference between supranuclear and intranuclear facial nerve palsy is as follows:

		Supranuclear	Infranuclear
1.	Forehead muscle movement	Intact	Total facial palsy
2.	Tongue movement	Impaired	Normal
3.	Ataxia	Present	No ataxia
4.	Associated hemiplagia	Present	Not present
5.	Tone	Maintained	Tone is flaccid
6.	Reflexes	Intact	Absent
7.	Muscle atrophy	No	Present
8.	Muscle fasciculation	Absent	Present

Glomus Tumors

CASE: A 42-year-old-female presented with history of deafness and tinnitus of incidious onset, slowly progressive in right ear for last 8 years.

She noticed polypoidal lesion in the ear and has occasionally blood-stained discharge since 10 months. History reveals that tinnitus is reduced by compression over the jugular vein in the neck. Examination of the ear reveals a mass in the external auditory canal.

Provisional Diagnosis: Glomus Tumor

Q.1 What is glomus tumor?
Ans. 1. It is benign, nonencapsulated, slow growing, locally invasive and vascular tumor arising from the glomus bodies (resembles carotid bodies) are present at dome of jugular bulb, hypotympanum, promontory and along the tympanic plexus, arising from the tympanic branch of IX nerve (Jacobson's nerve). It is also called chemodectoma because it resembles carotid bodies.
2. Blood supply: Jugulotympanic, tympanic branch of ascending pharyngeal artery.
3. The tumor arises from paraganglionic cells of neuroectoderm. These cells produce catecholamines and neuropeptides serving as a neurotransmitters.

Q.2 What is the age and sex relation in glomus tumor?
Ans. It is common in people between 40–50 years of age. It is five times more common in females.

Q.3 What are the characteristic histological features?
Ans. If contains three elements:
1. Epitheloid cells.
2. Vein and capillaries.
3. Connective tissue.
Epitheloid cells are found in plenty with large oval nuclei and granular cytoplasm are arranged either in the form of alveoli bordered by capillaries or in the form of cords. They may be arranged in groups

separated by fibrous tissue containing dilated veins. The veins does not have middle muscular layer. Paraganglioma are formed by cluster Zellballen chief cells.

Q.4 What are the various types of glomus tumor?

Ans. Type 1: Glomus tympanicus arises from promontory and confined to middle ear (Type I).

Type 2: Glomus jugulare arises from dome at jugular bulb and is limited to middle ear and bulb of jugular vein (Type II).

Type 3: Glomus jugular tumors : It destroys the bone and may invade the mastoid and petrous apex (Type III).

Type 4: Tumor extend into base of skull, middle ear and posterior cranial fossa. Jugular foramen with IX to XII cranial nerve may be involved.

Q.5 How glomus tumors are classified? (According to Oldring and Fisch)

Ans. According to Oldring and Fisch, classification of glomus tumor is as follows:

1. Type I: Localized to middle ear cleft.
2. Type II: Tympanomastoid tumors with no destruction of infralabyrinthine compartment.
3. Type III: Tumor involving infralabyrinthine region.
4. Type IV: Intracranial extension.

Q.6 What are the various clinical features of glomus tumor?

Ans. In 90% of cases symptoms are related to ear.

Clinical features may be grouped as follows:

1. Intratympanic group: In cases of tumor within middle ear with intact tympanic membrane. Earliest symptoms are:
   a. Conductive deafness is slowly progressive.
   b. Tinnitus: Early symptom is pulsatile and of swishing character, synchronous with pulse and can be temporarily stopped by carotid pressure. It is reduced by compression over jugular vein in the neck.
   c. Otoscopy: In initial stage a red reflex hue through intact TM in case of small tumor on promontory:
      – Rising sun appearance in case of tumor in hypotympanum
      – Later on pinkish mass behind the intact TM
      – Bluish appearance with bulging TM.
   d. On ear examination: Brown's sign (Pulsation sign) is positive, i.e. application of pressure over the tympanic membrane with the Seigle's speculum causes vigorously pulsation and then blanching and reverse happens with pressure release.
2. Tympanomastoid and ear polyp group:
   a. Tinnitus and deafness: Slowly progressive.
   b. Bleeding per ear: Scanty to profuse, spontaneously or on attempt to clean it.

    c. Dizziness is uncommon and indicates extension of disease into inner ear.

    d. Facial paralysis

    e. Ear ache: Less common

    f. Otorrhea: Due to secondary infection

    Examination reveals a red, vascular polypoidal mass filling the meatus. It bleeds readily and profusely on manipulation and biopsy.

3. Cranial nerve palsies group: In later stage after several years of ear symptoms, the tumor extends to involve the infralabyrinthine region and base of skull. It may spread over the mastoid or in the nasopharynx. IX to XII cranial nerve may be paralyzed. There may be dysphagia, hoarseness of voice, hypernasality and weakness of trapezius and sternomastoid muscles.

    Later on signs of intracranial extension may be present.

    Audible bruit: Auscultation with stethoscope over the mastoid region may reveal systolic bruit in all stages.

4. Systemic group: Some glomus tumor secretes catecholamine and produce various manifestations like headache, sweating, palpitation, hypertension, etc.

Q.7 What are the useful investigations in glomus tumor?

Ans. The useful investigations are: X-ray, CT scan, MRI, carotid angiography, jugular venography, lmpedance audiometry, blood for catecholamine level and urine for level of vanillylmandelic acid (VMA) or metanephrine level. Biopsy is avoided.

Q.8 What will be the findings in plain X-ray?

Ans. Plain X-ray (Jugular foramen view) shows expansion and erosion of jugular foramen.

Q.9 What are the findings in CT scan?

Ans. It is helpful in differentiating glomus tympanicum from glomus jugulare tumors. Caroticojugular spine (Crotch), i.e. bone between internal carotid artery and jugular vein is eroded in glomus jugulare tumor (Phelp's sign). It also helps to differentiate it from the aberrant carotid artery, high or dehiscent jugular bulb.

Q.10 What is the importance of MRI?

Ans. It demonstrate the soft tissue extent of tumor mass and delineates invasion of jugular bulb, vein, etc.

Q.11 What is four vessel angiography and its importance?

Ans. It is useful to find out extent of tumor, compression of internal carotid artery, and other associated carotid body tumor or embolization of the tumor. It is helpful in assessing brain perfusion study.

Q.12 What is the finding in impedence audiometry?

Ans. Oscillations in the impedance with the pulsations can be recorded.

Q.13 What is the treatment of glomus tumor?
Ans. 1. Radiotherapy in very elderly and inoperable tumor, residual or recurrence.
   2. Surgery is definitive treatment.
   3. Embolization to reduce vascularity: Preoperatively or in inoperable cases or following irradiation.

Q.14 What are the various surgical procedures done for glomus tumor?
Ans. Surgical procedure depends on the extent of tumor:
   1. Type A: Transmeatal approach and excision.
   2. Type B: Extended facial recess approach.
   3. Type C: Fisch infratemporal fossa approach (lateral approach).
   4. Type D: Skull-base approach and posterior fossa craniotomy.

Q.15 What is the differential diagnosis?
Ans. Differential diagnosis include malignant tumor, hemangioma, rhabdomyosarcoma, inflammatory polyp, malignant otitis external, osteomyillitis with granuloma, metastatic tumors from distant area like bronchus, breast, kidney, thyroid and prostate. Secondary tumor from adjacent area, e.g. nasopharynx, external meatus and the parotid.

Glass Cock-Jackson Classification

Classification of Glomus Tumor

Glomous Tympanicum

Type	Physical Findings
Type I	Small mass limited to promontory
Type II	Tumor completely filling middle ear space
Type III	Tumor filling middle ear and extending into mastoid process
Type IV	Tumor filling middle ear extending into mastoid process or through tympanic membrane to fill the external auditory canal. May extend anterior to internal carotid artery.

Glomus Jugulare

Type	Physical Findings
Type I	Small tumor involving jugular bulb, middle ear and mastoid process
Type II	Tumors extending under internal auditory canal, may have intracranial extension
Type III	Tumor extending in to petrous apex, may have intracranial extension
Type IV	Tumor extending beyond petrous apex into clivus as infratemporal fossa, may have intracranial extension

Presenting Sign and Symptoms

Among patients with glomus tumor

Sl. No.	Presenting symptoms	Glomus jugulare (n-106)	Glomus vagale (n-22)
	Pulsatile tinnitus	84=80	8=30
	Hearing loss	62=60	4=15
	Aural fullness	32=30	3=11
	Dysphagia	8=8	5=18
	Hoarseness of voice	12=11	4=15
	Vertigo	15=15	1=4
	Otalgia	13=12	3=12
	Facial weakness	15=15	1=4
	Ear bleeding	2=2	0
	Headache	5=5	0
	Dysartheria	0	0
	Pharyngeal fullness	0	9=4

SECTION 2

Head and Neck Diseases from ENT Perspective

⮞ Dermoid Cyst
⮞ Hemangioma
⮞ Lipoma
⮞ Capillary Hemangioma
⮞ Squamous Cell Carcinoma (Epithelioma)
⮞ Rodent Ulcer (Basal Cell Carcinoma)
⮞ Branchial Cyst
⮞ Branchial Fistula
⮞ Cystic Hygroma (Carvernous or Cystic Lmyphangioma)
⮞ Cervical Lymphadenitis
⮞ Thyroglossal Cyst
⮞ Ranula
⮞ Occult Primary with Neck Node (Metastasis)
⮞ Submandibular Sialoadenitis
⮞ Mixed Parotid Tumor (Pleomorphic Salivary Gland Tumor)
⮞ Malignant Tumor of Parotid Gland

Dermoid Cyst

CASE:
1. A spherical smooth surface soft, nonpulsalite, fluctuating swelling at postauricular region. Overlying skin is free and not adherent.
2. A spherical swelling of cherry size in the subcutaneous tissue at the inner angle of the eye (Fig. 1). The swelling is painless, slow growing, tense, fluctuating with smooth surface. It is not pulsatile and opaque with guttering of bone in the base underneath.

Provisional Diagnosis: Dermoid Cyst

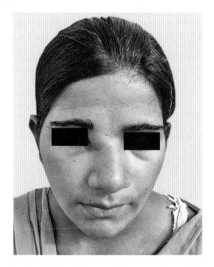

Fig. 1: A dermoid cyst at inner canthus of eye

Q.1 What is dermoid cyst?
Ans. 1. It is cyst located deep to skin and consists predominately of structure derived from primitive ectoderm.
2. It is cyst lined by squamous epithelium containing sebum, desquamated cell and sometimes hair and even teeth.

Q.2 What are different types of dermoid cyst?

Ans. Dermoid cyst can be:
1. Congenital:
   a. Sequestration dermoids
   b. Tubuloembryonic or tubulodermoids, e.g. thyroglossal cyst
2. Acquired:
   a. Implantion dermoids: Following puncturing wound in finger, palm, sole
   b. Teratomatous dermoids, e.g. ovary, testis.

Q.3 What is sequestration dermoids?

Ans. These are inclusion dermoids. These are found at sites of embryonic fusion and are due to inclusion of ectodermal layer in deeper tissue during process of closure of embryonic cleft and sinuses in the embryo. These may be noticed at birth or may be seen later in the life.

Q.4 What are the common sites of dermoids?

Ans. The common sites are:
1. Skull.
2. Inner canthus of the eye.
3. Outer canthus of the eye.
4. Postauricular.
5. Anterior triangle of the neck (Fig. 2).
6. Sublingual—median or lateral can be above myelohyoid muscle (Fig. 3) or below the myelohyoid muscle, can be bimanually palpable.
7. Midline at the root or dorsum of the nose.

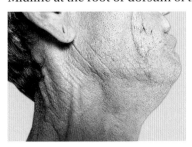 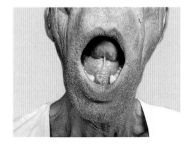

Fig. 2: Submandibular dermoid   **Fig. 3:** Sublingual dermoid

Q.5 Give points in favor of diagnosis.

Ans. The swelling is:
1. Painless, slow growing.
2. Situated at the line of embryonic fusion.
3. Skin over the swelling is free.
4. Soft in consistency, smooth.
5. Nonreducing, nonpulsatile.

Q. 6 What are common differential diagnosis?

Ans. 1. Sebaceous cyst: It is retention and distended cyst of sebaceous gland due to blockage of mouth, containing its own secretion (sebum) and desquamated epithelial cell.

2. Lipoma: Soft but noncystic and fluctuating.
3. Meningocele: Reducible and impulse on coughing.

Q.7 Why it is not sebaceous cyst?
Ans. It is not sebaceous cyst because it has:
1. No punctum.
2. Skin is free.
3. Deeper tissues are involved such as bone.

Q.8 What are complications if not treated.?
Ans. Complications are:
1. Infection.
2. Ulceration.
3. Pressure on deeper structure.

Q.9 What investigations are required?
Ans. X-ray of the local area is done (as these cyst causes bony indentition due to pressure) to see any gap at the base of cyst. In case of nasal dermoid, CT scan is done for any intracranial extension.

Q.10 What is treatment of dermoid cyst?
Ans. Enucleation with an appropriate incision (Fig. 4).

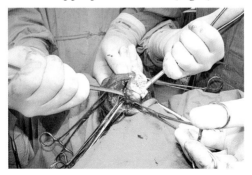

Fig. 4: Enucleation of the dermoid cyst

Q.11 What are defferences between dermoid cyst and sebaceous cyst?
Ans. The differences are:

Sl. No.	Sebaceous cyst	Dermoid cyst
1.	Adherent to skin	Skin is free
2.	Punctum: present	Absent
3.	Sebaceous material is expressed	Not
4.	Usually no hair	Hair may be present
5.	Lined by superficial cell	Lined by squamous cell epithelium
6.	Dose not indent the bone	Underlying bone is indented

Sublingual Dermoid

CASE: A painless, slow growing swelling in sublingual (Fig. 5) and submental region, it is smooth, soft, cystic in feel with free overlying skin and mucosa. It is opaque with guttering of mandible in the side.

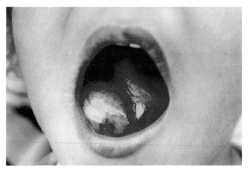

Fig. 5: Sublingual dermoid

Provisional Diagnosis: Sublingual Dermoid

Q.1 What is sublingual dermoid?
Ans. It is a sequestration dermoid arising due to inclusion of surface ectoderm (epithelial rests) in the midline at the fusion line of the mandibular arch.

Q.2 What are different types of sublingual dermoid?
Ans. According to site, they can be classified as:
1. Median sublingual dermoid either in floor of mouth or in submental region or both sides:
    a. Supramylohyoid—in the floor of mouth
    b. Infra- or submylohyoid—submental
2. Lateral (submandibular region):
    a. Supramylohyoid
    b. Submylohyoid.

Q.3 What are pathological features?
Ans. 1. Lining of the wall: Stratified squamous epithelium with or without dermal appendages.
    2. Contents: Doughy cheesy material and dose not contain hair unlike other dermoid cyst.

Q.4 What are clinical features?
Ans. 1. Visible swelling in the midline under the tongue (supramylohoid) or under the chin like double chin (inframylohoid).
    2. Freely mobile overlying skin or mucosa.
    3. Nontender and noncompressible.
    4. Spherical swelling with smooth surface.
    5. Edge cleanly defined.
    6. Limited mobility.

7. Soft and fluctuating.
8. Transillumination—negative.
9. Niether moves on deglutation nor on protruding of tongue.
10. Bimanually palpable.

Q.5 What are features of supramylohyoid variety?

Ans. On lifting tongue, the swelling mostly bulges intraorally but it bulges downwards in the submental region as mouth is closed and oral swelling compressed down by tongue.

Q.6 What are features of inframylohyoid varieties?

Ans. Midline cystic swelling bulges most prominently in the submental region looking like double chin. If the tongue is pushed up against the roof of mouth with teeth clenched, it bulges out below in the submental region.

Q.7 What is lateral sublingual dermoid?

Ans. It is a sequestration dermoid developed from the region of the first branchial pouch (below the Wharton's duct and lingual nerve and anterior to stylohyoid ligament. The submandibular gland is displaced backward with enlargement of dermoid.

Q.8 What are complications?

Ans. 1. Cosmetic problem.
2. Infection.
3. Difficulty in swallowing.
4. Difficulty in breathing.
5. Difficulty in articulation.

Q.9 What is treatment of median sublingual dermoid cyst?

Ans 1. Extraoral excision—by curved incision in the neck.
2. Intraoral approach—by a vertical midline incision.

Q.10 What is treatment of lateral sublingual dermoid?

Ans. 1. Intraoral approach—for small size cyst.
2. Extraoral—submandibular incision for large cyst.

Q.11 What are differential diagnoses?

Ans. 1. Ranula.
2. Ludwig's angina.
3. Ectopic thyroid.
4. Thyroglossal cyst.
5. Suprahyoid bursitis.
6. Sebaceous cyst.
7. Lipoma.
8. Hemangioma.
9. Cystic hygroma.

Hemangioma

CASE: The tongue is large in size and volume showing a bluish-colored localized spongy swelling, which is compressible and refill rapidly on withdrawal of pressure. It is not pulsatile.

Provisional Diagnosis: Cavernous Hemangioma of the Tongue

Q.1 What is hemangioma?
Ans. Hemangioma is a being tumor that occurs in the endothelial being of blood vessels. It is often found on the skin or internal organs. It is most common type of tumor found in children.

Q.2 What are the points in favor of the diagnosis?
Ans. Points in favor of the diagnosis:
1. Present since birth.
2. Slow growing.
3. Bluish in color.
4. Localized spongy swelling.
5. Compressible.
6. Nonpulsatile.

Q.3 What are the common sites?
Ans. 1. Skin—face, cheek, ears, nose (Fig. 1A).
2. Mucous membrane—lip (Fig. 1B), mouth, tongue (Fig. 1C).

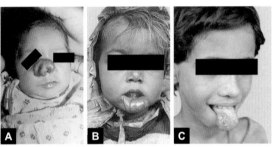

Figs 1A to C: (A) Hemangioma of the nose; (B) Hemangioma of the lip; (C) Hemangioma of the tongue

Q.4 What are the origins of hemangioma?

Ans. These may arise from:
1. Vein—cavernous hemangioma.
2. Artery—plexiform or arterial (Cirsoid aneurysm).
3. Capillary—capillary hemangioma.

Q.5 What are the diagnostic features of capillary hemangioma?

Ans. Capillary hemangioma:
1. Present since birth.
2. These are flat, red or purple patch.
3. Nonpulsatile.
4. Blanch on pressure.

Q.6 What are the diagnostic features of cirsoid aneurysm?

Ans. These are raised, pulsatile, partially compressible swelling with feeling of pulsating earth worms.

Q.7 What is the peculiarity of capillary hemangioma?

Ans. Majority of them disappears at the age of 8 years (not cavernous or arterial types).

Q.8 Which investigation is helpful?

Ans. Arteriography may help to detect the feeding vessels in large lesions.

Q.9 What is the treatment of cavernous hemangioma?

Ans. 1. Injection of sclerosing agents.
2. Cauterization.
3. Laser.

Q.10 What are the commonly used sclerosing agents?

Ans. 1. Boiling water.
2. Hypertonic solution.
3. Sodium morrhuate (3%).
4. Bleomycin (recently used).

Q.11 How is cautery done in cavernous hemangioma?

Ans. A needle is introduced into the lesion and is touched with diathermy. Thus, produced coagluation results in subsequent fibrosis.

Q.12 How does sclerosing agents effects?

Ans. Sclerosing agents produce fibrosis in the lesion and thereby obliterate the vascular spaces. Sclerosing treatment is usually done once a week up to 4-6 weeks, if required.

Q.13 What are complications of the hemangioma?

Ans. Various complications can occur if not treated. These are as follows:
1. Infection and septicemia.
2. Hemorrhage following trauma.
3. Ulceration.
4. Spontaneous coagulation.
5. Calcification (phlebolith).
6. Erosion of bone.

7. Arteriovenous fistula.
8. Angiosarcoma.

Q.14 Is there any role of surgery in cavernous hemangioma?
Ans. If the lesion is small and residual after sclerosing therapy, can be excised with diathermy.

Q.15 What happens if lesion is large and sclerosing treatment fails?
Ans. Arteriography is done to find the feeding arteries. The feeding vessels are then:
1. Ligated.
2. Embolization to oblilerate.
3. Excision.

Q.16 What are the common differential diagnosis of cavernous hemangioma?
Ans. 1. Dermoid cyst.
2. Neurofibroma.
3. Lipoma.

Lipoma

CASE: Slow-growing painless swelling in submandibular region (Fig. 1) which is smooth, lobulated, soft in consistency and mobile, overlying skin is free.

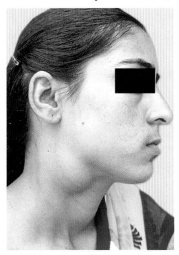

Fig. 1: Lipoma at submandibular region

Provisional Diagnosis: Lipoma

Q.1 What is lipoma?

Ans. It is a slow-growing encapsulated benign tumor of fat cell.

Q.2 What are points in favor of lipoma?

Ans. Points in favor are:

1. Slow growing swelling.
2. Painless.
3. Smooth and lobulated surface.
4. Soft and mobile.
5. Pseudofluctuation.
6. Margin slips under examining finger.
7. Covering skin is free

Q.3 What are the classical features of lipoma?
Ans. 1. Lobulated soft swelling.
2. Slipping of margin of the swelling under examining finger.

Q.4 How is lipoma classified?
Ans. 1. True lipoma is well-capsulated benign connective tissue tumor
2. Pseudolipoma is diffuse lipomatosis in which there is fatty infiltration of subcutaneous tissues, abdominal wall, neck, chin, etc.

Q.5 What are histological type of lipomas?
Ans. 1. Pure lipoma adipose tissue only.
2. Naevolipoma is mixed with hemangiomatous tissue.
3. Fibrolipoma contains excessive amount of fibrous tissue.
4. Neurolipoma contains nerve tissue.

Q.6 What is Dercum's disease?
Ans. Diffuse or nodular painfull deposits of fat in the neck, axilla, hips and thigh is called Dercum disease or adiposis dolorosa. It is associated with neurolipoma.

Q.7 Why does lipoma lobulated?
Ans. Subcutaneous fat is present in fibrous compartmcnts in lipoma. There is localized excessive accumulation of fat and they become prominent on surface, so become lobulated.

Q.8 What are the other conditions where "slip sign" may be positive?
Ans. Slip sign may be present in lymph node, and pericanalicular fibro-adenomas also.

Q.9 What is the utility of slip sign?
Ans. It is useful in differentiating solid encapsulated swelling from cystic swelling where the margin yields to pressure and does not slip.

Q.10 What are the complications in lipoma?
Ans. The complications are:
1. Myxomatous degeneration.
2. Calcification.
3. Fat necrosis due to repeated trauma.
4. Ulceration in the overlying skin due to repeatedly friction.
5. Sarcomatous change.

Q.11 What are the other conditions in differential diagnosis?
Ans. These are:
1. Fibroma.
2. Neurofibroma.
3. Fibrosarcoma.
4. Cold abscess.
5. Dermoid cyst.
6. Sebaceous cyst.
7. Hematoma.

8. Cystic hygroma,
9. Branchial cyst.

Q.12 What is the treatment of lipoma?
Ans. 1. Excision.
2. Liposuction.

Q.13 What are the peculiarities of lipoma?
Ans. The peculiarities are:
1. These are not usually found in children.
2. This is not neoplasm but a hamartoma or excessive accumulation.
3. Universal tumor can occur anywhere.
4. Commonly solitary, may be multiple.
5. Spread is finger-like process in subcutaneous spaces from lipoma.

Capillary Hemangioma

CASE: A sessile red swelling on the side of the nose, protruding from the skin surface since birth; the lesion is soft, compressible and mobile over the deep tissues.

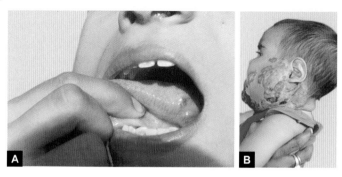

Figs 1A and B: (A) Hemangioma of the tongue; (B) Hemangioma at left parotid region

Provisional Diagnosis: Capillary Hemangioma

Q.1 What is capillary hemangioma?
Ans. It is a network of newly formed capillary-filled with blood. The blood chamber is very small and endothelial cells packed, so the lumen gets obliterated.

Q.2 What are the common sites?
Ans. 1. Skin—face (Fig. 1B), nose, lip and ear.
     2. Mucosa—nose, lip, tongue (Fig. 1A) and cheek.

Q.3 What are various types of capillary hemangioma?
Ans. 1. Strawberry naevus: A bright red lesion presents at birth, looks like a strawberry, arises from skin surface and sessile. The surface is irregular but covered with a smooth-pitted epithelium. It is compressible but not pulsatile. The lesion grows up to 1–2 years, then gradually get disappear with color fading and flattening process of the lesion up to the age of 7–8 years.

2. Portwine stain: Presents at birth and hardly changes in the life. It is a diffuse telangiectasia with no swelling. It is simple deep purple red-colored patch on the skin. The color can be diminished by local pressure.
3. Simple nevus: The lesion is a central red spot (due to dilated skin arterioles) with radical spreading small branches of feeding vessels giving an appearance of legs of a spider. The lesion is compressible and refill on release of pressure.

Q.4 What is treatment of capillary hemangioma?

Ans. 1. Strawberry naves: No treatment, it disappears at the age of 7–8 years (natural involution).
2. Portwine stain and spider naevus: Small lesion can be treated with carbon dioxide snow applied for 20 seconds at monthly interval. The dilated capillary gradually gets fibrosed. Large lesion should not be treated if not causing great cosmetic problem. Excision and skin grafting can be done. Laser beam therapy required.

Squamous Cell Carcinoma (Epithelioma)

CASE: Ulcer on the nose with raised, irregular and everted margin, with indurated hard base, the floor is covered with dirty slough with foul blood-stained discharge. It may be cauliflower in shape. Regional lymph node may be involved.

Provisional Diagnosis: Epithelioma

Q.1 What is provisional diagnosis?
Ans. Squamous cell carcinoma.

Q.2 What is squamous cell carcimoma?
Ans. It is carcinoma arising from prickle cell layer of epidermis, so it is also called epithelioma or epidermoid carcinoma.

Q.3 What are the points in favor of diagnosis?
Ans. 1. Ulcerative growth for the last 5 months with history of occasional bleeding.
2. Ulcer is circular 2 × 2 cm in size with raised and everted margin with indurated base, floor is having necrosed slough (Fig. 1).
3. Regional lymph nodes are enlarged.

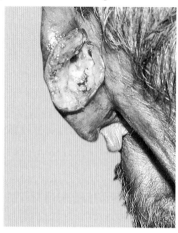

Fig. 1: Ulcerative growth on the medial surface of the pina

Q.4 Name the premalignant conditions if any?

Ans. 1. Long standing ulcers following burns (Marjolin's ulcer), venous ulcer.
   2. Leukoplakia.
   3. Senile keratosis.

Q.5 What are the common sites of epithelioma?

Ans. 1. Anywhere on the skin, mainly exposed parts.
   2. At the junction of skin and mucous membrane, e.g. lip, nasal vestibule.
   3. The part which are lined by squamous epithelium, e.g. tongue, oral cavity, pharynx, larynx, esophagus.
   4. Following metaplasia of epithelium:
      a. Columnar epithelium—nasal cavity, sinuses.
      b. Transitional epithelium—nasopharynx.

Q.6 What are the common differential diagnosis?

Ans. The lesion is to be differentiated from:
   1. Basal cell carcinoma.
   2. Melanoma mainly a melanotic.
   3. Pilometrioma.
   4. Oriental sore.

Q.7 What are the common routes of spread?

Ans. Direct and lymphatic spread are common but hematogenous spread can also occur.

Q.8 Describe the histological features?

Ans. Epithelial pearls or cell nest is classical feature. Epithelial pearls are masses of keratin surrounded by prickle cells in concentric or onion skin. Epithelial pearl is absent in squamous cell carcinoma of esophagus because keratin formation from prickle cell layer of skin is not seen in this area.

Q.9 What is the line of treatment?

Ans. Surgery or radiotherapy.

Rodent Ulcer
(Basal Cell Carcinoma)

CASE: An ulcer on the nose involving tip and part of dorsum extending lateral side to involve the part of ala, it is superficial, red in colour, at places covered with a scab, removal of scab cause slight bleeding. Edge is slightly raised, irregular and beaded. Regional lymph nodes are not enlargard.

Provisional Diagnosis: Rodent Ulcer

Q.1 What is possible diagnosis of the ulcer?
Ans. It is a basal cell carcinoma, i.e. rodent ulcer.

Q.2 What is a rodent ulcer?
Ans. It is locally-invasive carcinoma arising from the basal layer of epidermis.

Q.3 What are the points in favor of diagnosis?
Ans. Several points favoring the diagnosis are:
1. Painful ulcerative growth at the dorsum of the nose with occasional itching and bleeding.
2. The lesion is situated on the face just in an area where basal cell carcinoma occurs.
3. Ulcer is about 1.5 × 2 cm size, edge is raised irregular and beaded (rolled).
4. Regional lymph node not enlarged.

Q.4 What is the common site of a rodent ulcer?
Ans. It is commonly found on the face above a line drawn from the angle of mouth to the lobule of the ear. The part which is exposed to ultraviolet irradiation (bright sunlight).
Common sites are:
1. Around the inner canthus of eye.
2. Around the outer canthus of eye.
3. Nose.
4. Ear and around it.

Q.5 Why is it called rodent ulcer?

Ans. The lesion spreads mainly by direct invasion, i.e. destroying and eroding the surrounding tissue or burrows the underlying tissue deeply like rodent, so it is called rodent ulcer. Lymphatic or hematogenous spread does not occur.

Q.6 What are the etiological factors?

Ans. It is common in:
1. Elderly people.
2. Males.
3. White skinned people.
4. Exposure to sun.

Q.7 What are different clinical types of rodent ulcer?

Ans. Different types are:
1. Ulcerative: Edge is raised, irregular and beaded (Fig. 1B)
2. Nodular: Starts as a nodule, smooth, glistening and translucent like pearly white nodule under the epidermis (Fig. 1A). Surface is covered with fine blood vessels. Nodule may finally ulcerate.
3. Cystic: It is a variety of nodular which does not ulcerate. It attain quite large size and look like cyst. Actually it is not cystic because it is solid and nonfluctuant.
4. Field-fire or geographical: Advancing edge with healing central area consisting of flat white scar.
5. Basi-squamous: Rarely the ulcer takes on a squamous cell carcinomatous change giving rise to mixed appearance of a basal cell and squamous cell carcinoma.

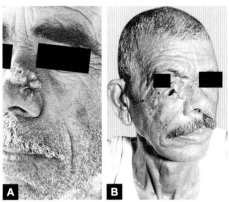

Figs 1A and B: (A) Nodular variety of basal cell carcinoma; (B) Ulcerative lesion of the skin of the face

Q.8 What is differential diagnosis?

Ans. 1. It should be differentiated from squamous cell carcinoma, malignant melanoma, keratoacanthoma, pyogenic granuloma and cutaneous oriental sore.

2. In squamous cell carcinoma, history is of short duration only a few month, the lesion can occur in any part of the skin, which may be as nodule or a fungating ulcer with bleeding tendency on touch and with raised and everted margin or a cauliflower mass. Regional lymph nodes are enlarged.

3. In malignant melanoma, the lesion arises (in about 50% of cases) from a preexisting naevi. The ulcer is dark coloured, no rolled up edge. Regional lymph nodes are enlarged. Satellite nodules are present.

4. Keratoacanthoma is a self-limiting overgrowth and subsequent necrosis of a sebaceous gland with a short history of a few weeks. The lesion starts as a nodule with central sloughing and does not extend to the surrounding tissue. Spontaneous regression occurs.

5. Pyogenic granuloma appears as soft red nodules with very short history of few days. It bleeds easily till it heals and covered by skin or epithelial lining.

Q.9 How is the diagnosis confirmed?
Ans. Diagnosis is confirmed by incisional biopsy from growth.

Q.10 What is treatment of a rodent ulcer?
Ans. 1. Surgery.
2. Radiotherapy.
3. Cryosurgery.
4. Local 5FU cream.
5. Laser surgery.

Q.11 Indication of radiotherapy?
Ans. All cases can be treated but the lesion which is not close to eye and not fixed to bone is real indication.

Q.12 When surgery is indicated?
Ans. 1. If the lesion is very close to the eye.
2. If it is fixed to bone.
3. Recurrence after radiotherapy.

Q.13 What is the principle of excision?
Ans. Three-dimensional excision with 3 mm normal tissue margin followed by closure of defect with any of the following:
1. Direct suture.
2. Skin grafting.
3. Pedicle grafts.
4. Rotation flaps.

Q.14 Describe the microscopic features of rodent ulcer.
Ans. The lesion shows cells in palisade (fence or guard wall) arrangement whereas the epithelioma shows keratin or epithelial pearl.

Branchial Cyst

CASE: Cystic ovoid swelling behind the anterior edge of the upper third of sternomastoid muscle (Fig. 1). Its long axis is forward and downward.

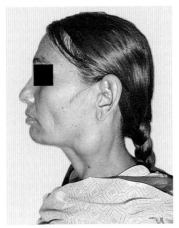

Fig. 1: Branchial cyst

Provisional Diagnosis: Branchial Cyst

Q.1 What are the points in favor of diagnosis?
Ans. 1. Patient is an adolescent adult.
   2. Painless swelling in upper and lateral part of the neck (Fig. 1) for 3 years duration.
   3. Situated on anterior border at junction of upper one-third and lower two-third of the sternomastoid muscle.
   4. It is ovoid 3 × 3 in size with smooth surface, well-defined margin and soft cystic in feel.
   5. Negative transillumination, restricted mobility, not compressible.
   6. Regional lymph node: Not enlarged.

Q.2 What are other features?
Ans. It is congenital abnormality but usually get notice near puberty or later on in early adult life as fluid collection in cyst takes a prolonged course.

Q.3 What is the origin of branchial cyst?

Ans. The growth of the second branchial arch is much rapid then that of the arches below, so that it soon overhangs them forming a deep groove called the cervical sinus. Ridges from overgrown second and fifth branchial arch fuse to close the space (cervical sinus). It disappears entirely. If this space persists (which is lined by squamous epithelium), fluid gradually collects in it and branchial cyst is thus formed.

Q.4 What is the peculiarity of cystic fluid?

Ans. The fluid is thick golden-yellow in color and shimmers with fat globules. It contains cholesterol crystals (Dental cyst and dentigerous cyst also contain cholesterol crystal).

Q.5 What is the relation of neck structures to branchial cyst?

Ans. It is superficial to structure derived from the third arch, i.e. internal carotid artery, the glossopharyngeal nerve, and sternopharyngeal muscle. Deep to structures derived from the second arch, i.e. the lesser cornu of the hyoid bone, stylohyoid ligament, stylohyoid and posterior belly of the digastric muscles, the facial nerve and the external carotid artery.

Q.6 What are the complications of branchial cyst?

Ans. 1. Recurrent infection (in the lymphoid tissue in its wall) when it become painful so restricted neck movement and opening of mouth.

2. Abscess may be mistaken for simple abscess and drain thus discharging sinus in the upper neck results. It is called acquired branchial fistula.

Q.7 What are common differential diagnosis?

Ans. 1. Cervical lymph node enlargement: Solid swelling multiple in number.

2. Cold abscess: Matted lymph nodes at the base. Not transparent. Aspirated content is tubercular pus.

3. Submandibular gland swelling situated at a higher level in submandibular triangle.

4. Carotid body tumor situated beneath the anterior edge of the sternomastoid muscle at the level of the carotid bifurcation. The swelling is solid, hard and dull on percussion. It is pulsatile, can move horizontally but not up and down. It may bulge into the oropharynx (lateral wall) bruit is present.

Q.8 What is the treatment of branchial cyst?

Ans. Complete excision through a collar incision.

Q.9 What precautions will you take during excision?

Ans. 1. Complete removal of cyst wall if small portion—left, it recur.

2. The nerves deep to cyst must be protected are:
   a. Hypoglossal nerve.
   b. Glossopharyngeal nerve.
   c. Spinal accessory nerve.

Branchial Fistula

CASE: Child having a discharging sinus situated at lower third of the neck at anterior border of sternomastoid muscle.

Provisional Diagnosis: Branchial Fistula

Q.1 What are the points in favor of your diagnosis?

Ans. The points in favor of diagnosis are:
1. Discharging sinus in the lower third of the neck at anterior border of sternomastoid muscle (Fig. 1A).
2. Fistula has a well-defined margin above, surrounding skin shows excoriation. Fistula is covered with a scab.
3. Discharge is watery, glairy or mucopurulent.
4. On swallowing, opening of the tract goes inwards causing a dimple. Due to pulling or puckering in case of complete fistula.
5. Deglutation makes the skin opening more prominent.

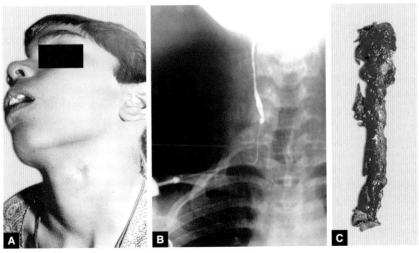

Figs 1A to C: (A) Branchial fistula; (B) Sinogram of branchial fistula; (C) Excised specimen of branchial fistula

Q.2 Is it congenital or acquired?

Ans. It may be congenital or acquired. This can be diagnosed by its site:
1. Congenital is at lower third of the neck.
2. Acquired is at upper third of the neck.

Q.3 Where does the fistula tract open?

Ans. It is subcutaneous up to thyroid cartilage then it pierces deep fascia and passes through two branches of carotid arteries. It passes deep to posterior belly of digastric and passes superficial to hypoglossal nerve, internal jugular vein and opens into posterior pillar of fauces behind the tonsil. In most cases, the tract cannot reach up to the pharynx.

Q.4 What is the origin of branchial cyst?

Ans. It arises as a result of partial failure of fusion between the second and fifth arches.

Q.5 How does the origin of a branchial fistula differ from thyroglossal fistula?

Ans. Branchial fistula can either be congential or acquired, but thyroglossal fistula is always acquired.

Q.6 How the fistulous tract is assessed?

Ans. 1. X-ray taken after preoperative injection of a radiopaque dye through its external orifice (sinogram) as shown in Figure 1B.
2. Ultrasonography.
3. MRI.
4. Injection of methylene blue on the operation table.

Q.7 What is the treatment of branchial fistula?

Ans. Excision of fistula by step-ladder pattern of dissection (Fig. 1C).

Q.8 What is branchial sinus?

Ans. It is incomplete branchial fistula. It is blind internally as it is obliterated on the lateral pharyngeal wall but shows only an external opening.

Q.9 Describe the wall and lining of the fistula.

Ans. The tract enclosed by muscles and lined by:
1. External part up to cleft membrane by squamous epithlium.
2. Internal part by columnar epithelium (may be destroyed by recurrent infection).

Cystic Hygroma (Cavernous or Cystic Lymphangioma)

CASE: A child with multiloculated cystic swelling in the posterior triangle. It is lobulated, brilliantly transparent, partially compressible.

Provisional Diagnosis: Cystic Hygroma

Q.1 What is cystic hygroma?

Ans. It is a collection of lymphatic sacs which is lined by an endothelial layer. It contains clear colorless lymph. It is a cavernous lymphangioma or cystic lymphangioma, with wide ramifications. It is congenital malformation (hamartoma) affecting lymphatic channel.

Q.2 What are sites of cystic hygroma?

Ans. 1. In the neck: Usually at the base of the posterior triangle.
2. Other sites: The cheek, axilla, mediastinum, groin, mouth. Occasionally in breast, parotid region.

Q.3 How does it originate in the neck?

Ans. It is due to sequestration of portion of a jugular lymph sac (primitive lymph sac) from the lymphatic system in mesoblast one on each side, between internal jugular vein and subclavian veins, during embryonic life.

Q.4 What is the age for manifestation of cystic hygroma?

Ans. 1. At birth.
2. Soon after birth.
3. Mostly during the first year of life.
4. Young children.
5. Rarely in the adult life.

Q.5 What is gross pathological features?

Ans. 1. Multilobulated and multilocular, thin-walled cystic mass in the subcutaneous tissue.
2. A collection of cyst-like mass of soap-bubbles, having larger cysts near the surface and deeper smaller cyst tend to lesser extend out- along facial planes, between nerve and vessels and even infiltrates the muscle fibers and nerves.

3. Cysts communicates directly or indirectly with each other.
4. Cut surface is haphazardly honey combed.

Q.6 What are common presenting features?

Ans. Parent complaints of:
1. Lump in the neck.
2. Disfigurement.

Q.7 What are characteristic features of swelling of cystic hygroma?

Ans. 1. Swelling: Usually presents in posterior triangle, enlarges upward towards the ear and sometimes supraclavicular and spreads in one side of the neck (Fig. 1). It may even extend into the mediastinum.
2. It visibly increases in size when the child strains.
3. Surface in lobulated, lying in subcutaneous tissue with ill-defined margins.
4. Overlying skin is free and normal in texture. Sometimes it has a bluish tinge in it.
5. It is cystic, soft and partially compressible like a fluid-filled sponge (due to intercommunicated cysts).
6. Dull on percussion.
7. Brilliantly transparent.
8. Mostly, is superficial but sometimes it may be partly deep to sternomastoid muscle.
9. No cervical lymph node enlargement.

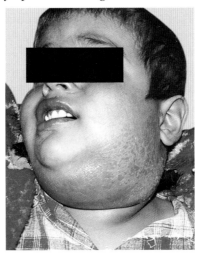

Fig. 1: Neck swelling (cystic hygroma)

Q.8 What are the complications?

Ans. Complications are:
1. Recurrent infection
2. Respiratory distress (due to sudden increase in size)
3. Lymphorrhoe—if ruptures
4. Obstruction of labor if present at birth.

Q.9 What is its fate or termination?

Ans. Spontaneous recovery is a possibility and takes about 2 years.

Q.10 What investigations should be done?

Ans. 1. X-ray chest: To exclude mediastinal extension.

2. CT scan or MRI: To assess the exact extent of the lesion and its relation to vital structures.

Q.11 What is the treatment?

Ans. 1. Can be observed for 1–2 years for spontaneous regression if not causing life-threatening problem or not rapidly enlarging.

2. Preoperative sclerosant solution injection (hypertonic saline or boiling water) into the cysts. It may be benificial:
   a. Decrease in size.
   b. Fibrosing the cyst wall.
   c. Swelling becomes localized.
   d. Easy to operate.

4. Excision (wide exposure): Should be complete as far as possible.

5. Incomplete excision: If not possible: It can be done in case of nerve involvement and other problems.

Q.12 What are differential diagnosis?

Ans. 1. Pneumatocele (aerocele).

2. Pharyngeal pouch.

3. Hemangioma.

4. Branchial cyst.

5. Lipoma.

CASE

26

Cervical Lymphadenitis

CASE: Slowly-progressive swellings in the upper part of lateral side of neck which are matted and mildly painful. There is an opening in the center of a few mass over which the skin is thin and mildly bluish.

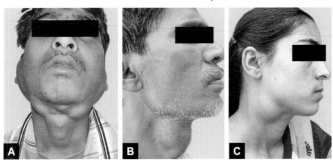

Figs 1A to C: Showing lymph-node enlargement at different sites

Provisional Diagnosis: Tuberculous Cervical Lymphadenitis with Cold Abscess of Jugulodigastric Lymph Nodes

Q.1 What are points in favor of tuberculosis?
Ans. 1. Swelling consists of matted deep cervical group of lymph node in the upper lateral side of neck.
   2. There may be softening at the center of few swellings (formation of cold abscess).
   3. Swelling has no sign of acute inflammation (Figs 1B and C).
   4. Swelling is of one year duration.

Q.2 What other features can occur in tuberculous lymphadenitis?
Ans. Other presentations may be:
   1. Cold abscess.
   2. Ulcer with thin-undermined edge with bluish pigmentation of the surrounding skin; with pale granulation tissue in the floor with slight induration at the base.
   3. Sinus formation with thin margin and undermined edge with serosanguinous discharge.

Q.3 How does tuberculous infection reach these lymph nodes ?

Ans. 1. By lymphatics either from pharynx usually tonsils or teeth to upper cervical lymph nodes or from the lung to the mediastinal nodes to lower cervical group.

2. By blood stream from any tuberculous focus in the body.

Q.4 What are the characteristic differences when it spreads?

Ans. 1. A localized group of lymph nodes is involved if infection spreads by lymphatic route.

2. The initial tubercles in lymphatic route are the lymph sinus around the periphery of lymph node. In blood-borne infection, the lymph nodes are generalized or irregularly affected and general systemic manifestations like weakness, cough, fever, etc. are common. Earlier lesion is central in lymph node.

Q.5 Which group of glands is commonly involved?

Ans. Jugulodigastric lymph nodes are commonly involved.

Q.6 What is lymphatic drainage of head and neck?

Ans. It can be classified into two forming groups:

1. Regional group (circular chain)
2. Terminal group (vertical chain of deep cervical nodes)
   a. The regional group is classified according to the region drained, (1) Occipital; (2) Mastoid (retroauricular); (3) Parotid on or within parotid gland; (4) Buccal (facial) on buccinator muscle; (5) Submandibular; (6) Submental; (7) Anteriocervical—along the course of anterior jugular vein; (8) Superficial cervical along the course of external jugular vein; (9) Laryngeal (Delphian)—on the cricopharyngeal ligament; (10) Tracheal, pretracheal and paratracheal; (11) Supraclvicular.
   b. Terminal group (vertical chain of deep cervical nodes) closely related to carotid sheath and in particular to internal jugular vein and receives all the lymphatics via one of the regional groups. There are: (1) Upper deep; (2) Middle deep; (3) Lower deep cervical. Two of the nodes of deep cervical nodes are: (a) Jugulodigastric node: situated about ½ to 1 cm below the angle of mandible. It lies just below the posterior belly of diagastric muscle where it crosses the jugular vein. It mainly drains the tonsil and tongue; (b) Jugulo-omohyoid node: It lies at the crossing of internal jugular vein with the intermediate tendon of omohyoid muscle. It mainly drains the tongue. The efferent lymph vessels from deep cervical chain, join to form the jugular lymph trunk. This vessel drains into thoracic duct or right lymphatic duct. Alternatively, it may drain into the subclavian trunk or independently into bracheocephalic vein.

Q.7 What is the differential diagnosis?

Ans. 1. For the solid lymph nodes:
   – Chronic nonspecific lymphadenitis
   – Lymphoma

- Secondaries
- Carotid body tumor.
2. Cystic swelling (cold abscess):
 - Branchial cyst
 - Antibioma.
3. With a sinus:
 - Acquired branchial fistula
 - Actinomycosis.

Q.8 What are the stages of tubercular cervical lymphadenitis?

Ans. The stages of tubercular cervical lymphadenitis are:
1. Stage of discrete lymph node enlargement: The lymph nodes are enlarged, discrete, painless as caseating necrosis has occurred in the gland.
2. Stage of matting: Due to development of periadenitis, lymph nodes become adherent together and matting occurs.
3. Stage of cold abscess: Pus is formed in the gland which turns into cold abscess.
4. Stage of ulcer formation or sinus development: Pus penetrates the deep fascia and comes superficially to form a discharging sinus on the surface.

Q.9 What is the histological picture of tuberculous lymphadenitis?

Ans. A homogeneous, caseous centre, staining red with eosin, a periphery of pale epitheloid cells with one or more Langhan's giant cells and outer zone of lymphocytes and fibroblasts.

Q.10 Describe Langhan's giant cells and how do they differ from ordinary cells?

Ans. 1. Langhan's giant cells are formed by fusion of a number of epitheloid cells. They attain a great size and contain a large number of nuclei, usually arranged either around the periphery or at one or both the poles like garland. The center of the cell is necrotic.
2. Ordinary foreign body giant cells contain small nuclei scattered throughout the cytoplasm.

Q.11 What are the pathological varieties of tuberculous lymphadenitis?

Ans. The pathological varieties are:
1. The lymphadenoid or proliferative form: Hyperplasia of the lymphoid tissue and little caseation. The capsule remains unbroken and nodes are discrete.
2. Fibrous variety: Little caseation or lymphoid hyperplasia. The lymph node shows a progressive fibrosis. Common in adults (senile form).
3. The caseating form: Common in children. Foci of caseation is enlarge and coalesce to a cold abscess.

Q.12 Why it is called cold abscess?

Ans. An infected lymph node caseates and turn into pus. The procedure is very slow and does not stimulate excessive hyperemia. So skin temperature is normal, therefore, called as cold abscess. Due to waxy sheath around the bacilli, necrosis to the tissue is less than the surface of rapidly multiplying bacteria (pyogenic), so the type of cellular response is less acute.

Q.13 What is the collar-stud abscess?

Ans. A tubercular abscess penetrates deep fascia and comes superficially into subcutaneous tissue. It has two compartments, one on either side of the deep fascia connected by small central tract.The shape resembles a collar-stud, hence, it is called as collar-stud abscess.

Q.14 What investigations are needed to be done?

Ans. Main investigations are:
1. Blood for TLC, DLC and ESR.
2. X-ray chest PA view for lung lesion.
3. Mantoux test.
4. Pus culture and smear for AFB.
5. FNAC.
6. Sputum examination for AFB.
7. Excisional biopsy.

Q.15 What is the treatment of cervical lymphadenitis?

Ans. The treatment include:
1. Antitubercular drugs for 9–12 months
2. Cold abscess repeated aspiration
3. Residual lymph node excision.

Metastatic Lymph Node Neck

CASE: A hard (often stony), nontender, smooth large mass, fixed in the neck (Fig. 2).

Provisional Diagnosis: Metastatic Cervical Lymphadenopathy

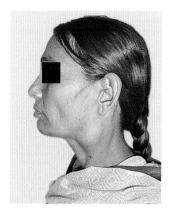

Fig. 2: Submandibular lymph node metastasis

Q.1 What are local features of metastatic nodes?

Ans. 1. Lymph nodes are hard (often stony) nontender, smooth or irregular, discrete or a large mass.
   2. These may be mobile in transverse direction or fixed (tumor spread beyond the capsule of the nodes).
   3. Overlying skin free with normal color or fixed in advanced cases (skin is pale or blotchy red).

Q.2 What is the pattern of secondary lymph node metastasis in neck?

Ans. Levels of lymphatic pattern are:
   1. Submental and submandibular.
   2. Upper jugular (Fig. 2)
   3. Middle jugular
   4. Lower jugular
   5. Posterior compartment
   6. Anterior compartment
   7. Upper mediastinal nodes.

Q.3 What are the common sites of primary?

Ans. Common sites are:
   1. Oral cavity
   2. Pharynx—oro, naso, hypo
   3. Larynx
   4. Lung
   5. Thyroid.

Q.4 What are the possible sites of affected node?

Ans. Crudely possible sites of the primary are:
   1. Lesion above hyoid—upper deep cervical node.
   2. Larynx and thyroid—middle and lower deep cervical node.
   3. Intrabdominal, thoracic and testes—supraclavicular node (Virchow's node).

Q.5 What are the investigations to detect site of primary carcinoma.

Ans. Investigations are:
   1. Clinical history.
   2. Clinical examination of ENT and head and neck region.
   3. Direct laryngoscopy and biopsy.
   4. Barium swallow.
   5. X-ray chest PA view.
   6. Bronchoscopy and esophagoscopy.

Q.6 Some basic facts for secondary lymph node?

Ans. Tumors other than squamous cell carcinoma which metastasize to cervical lymph nodes are thyroid carcinoma, skin tumors and salivary gland tumors.

Q.7 What is staging of metastatic cervical lymph node?

Ans. Staging as:

    N-0 No regional lymph node metastasis.

    N-1 Metastasis in a single ipsilateral node (3 cm or less in greatest diameter).

    N-2a Ipsilateral single lymph node (3–6 cm in diameter).

    N-2b Ipsilateral multiple lymph nodes (not more than 6 cm in greatest diameter).

    N-2c Bilateral or contralateral lymph node (not more than 6 cm in greatest diameter).

    N-3 Lymph node greater than 6 cm in diameter.

Q.8 When does biopsy required?

Ans. 1. Primary is not found

      2. Node appears to be lymphoma

      3. Clinical or cytological (FNAC) uncertainity exists.

Q.9 Describe the policy of treatment?

Ans. 1. Classical radical neck dissection with excision of primary.

      2. Modified radical neck dissection.

      3. Functional neck dissection.

      4. Supraomohyoid neck dissection.

      5. Anterior neck dissection.

Lymphoma

CASE: Multiple cervical nodes are enlarged, nontender, discrete and soft (rubbery in consistency) (Fig. 1A).

Provisional Diagnosis: Lymphoma

Q.1 What are the points in favor of lymphoma (Hodgkin's disease)?

Ans: Points in favor are:

    1. Large discrete, nontender lymph nodes, soft to firm rubbery in consistency.

    2. Paul-Ebstein fever.

    3. Spleen and liver are enlarged.

    4. Eosinophilia.

Q.2 What are main types of lymphoma and what are the differences between the two?

Ans. Lymphoma is of two types mainly—Hodgkin's lymphoma and non-Hodgkin's lymphoma. The differences between two are as follows:

Hodgkin's lymphoma	Non-Hodgkin's lymphoma
1. Localized to groups of lymph nodes, such as cervical, axillary, inguinal are enlarged.	1. Multiple peripheral lymph nodes are enlarged.
2. Axial lymph nodes are involved, e.g. mediastinal, para-aortic.	2 Nonaxial lymph node are involved like peripheral Waldeyer's lymph node, Peyer's patch.
3. Extranodal or organ involved is 10%.	3. Involvement of organs is 40%.
4. Systemic features are not common.	4. Systemic features are common.
5. Matting of nodes is not common.	5. Matting is common and early.

Q.3 What are the histological characteristics of Hodgkin's lymphoma?

Ans. Lesion shows cellular infiltration of node with lymphocytes, histiocytes, eosinophils, Reed-Steinberg giant cells and fibrous tissue.

Q.4 What is Reed-Sternberg cell?

Ans. The nucleus is bilobed (mirror-imaged nuclei) due to division but cytoplasm does not divides. It is also found in infectious mononucleosis and other lymphoma.

Q.5 What are the different types of Hodgkin's lymphoma?

Ans. Hodgkin's lymphoma are:
  a. Lymphatic predominance.
  b. Mixed cellularity.
  c. Nodular sclerosis.
  d. Lymphocytic depletion.

Q.6 What are the different types of non-Hodgkin's lymphoma?

Ans. 1. Nodular:
     a. Lymphocytic
     b. Mixed
     c. Hisieocytic.
  2. Diffuse:
     a. Lymphocytic
     b. Mixed
     c. Histiocytic
     d. Lymphoblastic
     e. Burkitt's lymphoma.

Q.7 What are the investigations?

Ans. 1. X-ray chest—mediastinal enlargement.
  2. CT-scan—chest, abdomen, pelvis.

3. USG abdomen.
4. Lymph node biopsy.

Q.8 What are the clinical types of staging in Hodgkin's lymphoma?

Ans. Clinical staging are:
1. Stage I: Single lymph node region or single extralymphatic organ.
2. Stage II: Two or more lymph node region on one side of diaphragm.
3. Stage III: Lymph node on both the sides of diaphragm.
   a. Systemic features absent.
   b. Systemic features present.
4. Stage IV: Multiple or disseminated involvement of lymph nodes or organs.

Q.9 What is the treatment?

Ans. 1. Stage I, II, IIIA: Radiotherapy.
2. Stage IIIB: Chemotherapy + Radiotherapy.
3. Stage IV: Chemotherapy.

Q.10 What is the prognosis after treatment?

Ans. Five-year survival chances are as follows:
1. Stage I and II: 90%
2. Stage IIIA: 75%
3. Stage IIIB and IV: 50%

Q.11 Which histological type carries the best prognosis?

Ans. Lymphocytic predominance.

27

Thyroglossal Cyst

CASE: A small nodular swelling in the upper part of the neck, below the hyoid bone in the midline with smooth surface tense cystic to firm in consistency (positive fluctuation and Paget's test). The swelling moves up with deglutition and with protrusion of tongue (Figs 1A and B).

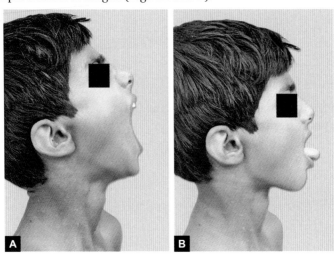

Figs 1A and B: (A) Midline swelling in upper part of neck;
(B) Swelling moves up with protrusion of tongue

Provisional Diagnosis: Thyroglossal Cyst

Q.1 What is thyroglossal cyst?
Ans. It is actually a tubular dermoid cyst arising from persistent thyroglossal duct.

Q.2 What is thyroglossal duct?
Ans. From the region of foramen caecum in early stage of fetal life, downward growth of solid column of cells take place which extends as far as upper border of thyroid cartilage. It crosses the region where the future hyoid bone is located and descends further downward to from pyramidal lobe

of thryoid. Later on this whole tract disappears. Occasionally it persists as a columnar epithelial lined tract after canalization.

Q.3 How does the thyroglossal tract or duct form the cyst?

Ans. Persistence of any part of the tract or duct may form a cystic swelling due to collected secretion. This cyst is called thyroglossal cyst.

Q.4 What are the anomalies of thyroglossal duct?

Ans. 1. Thyroglossal cyst and fistula.
     2. Accessory thyroid and ectopic thyroid.

Q.5 What is course of thyroglossal duct?

Ans. From the region of foramen cecum, it passes down in the midline through genioglossus muscles, geniohyoid muscles and then between two mylohyoid muscles and comes in close relation with the central part of body of the hyoid bone.

At the level of the hyoid bone it may either:
a. Pass in front of central part of hyoid bone.
b. Traverse the hyoid bone.
c. Hook behind the hyoid bone.

From the hyoid bone it comes down to the upper border of thyroid cartilage and to continue up to the pyramidal lobe or isthmus of thyroid gland. Thyroid follicles are found in one third of the specimens of thyroglossal duct remnant.

Q.6 What are the sites of thyroglossal cyst?

Ans. This varies with persistent of tract and may occur anywhere along the tract.
     1. Subhyoid—commonest.
     2. Suprahyoid.
     3. Overcricoid.
     4. Over thyroid cartilage.
     5. Floor of the mouth.
     6. Just below foramen cecum.

Q.7 Is it always present in the midline?

Ans. It usually occupies midline except in the region of thyroid cartilage where the thyroglossal tract is pushed to one side, usually to left.

Q.8 What are the contents of the cyst?

Ans. Transparent jelly-like material with cholesterol crystals.

Q.9 What are clinical features of thyroglossal cyst?

Ans. 1. Age: Common between 15 and 30, but can appear at any age.
     2. Painless swelling: In the midline neck.
     3. Oval swelling with long axis in the long axis of the neck.
     4. Overlying skin is free and normal.
     5. Smooth surface with well-defined margin
     6. Fluctuation is positive.

7. Transillumination test: Usually negative (because contents is thick due to desquamated epithelial cells or debris of past infection).
8. It can move side by side but not up and down.
9. Moves with deglutition (attached to hyoid bone with fibrous tissue).
10. Moves on protrusion of the tongue (due to connection of base of tongue to the cyst by duct fibrous remnants).
11. Positive tugging sensation—catch hold the cyst between the thumb and fore finger and ask the patient to deglutate, the cyst is tugged upwards.
12. Upward movement on protrusion may be absent if cyst lies below the level of thyroid cartilage.

Q.10 What are the complications?
Ans. 1. Recurrent infection: Swelling becomes painful, increases in size and become tender.
2. Fistula.

Q.11 What is the differential diagnosis?
Ans. 1. Adenoma in thyroid.
2. Sublingual dermoid.
3. Aberrant thyroid.
4. Enlarged lymph node.

Q.12 What is the treatment?
Ans. Sistrunk's operation: Complete extirpation of the thyroglossal tract with removal of a portion of the body of the hyoid bone.

Q.13 What are the other peculiarities of thyroglossal cyst?
Ans. 1. There are lymphoid tissue in the wall so infection is common.
2. If it hyoid bone is not excised, it recur.
3. Cyst wall contains thyroid tissue. Sometimes these tissues may be the only thyroid tissue acting as thyroid gland. Thyroid scan should be done before operation.

Thyroglossa Fistula

CASE: A small persistent sinus below the hyoid with glairy mucoid discharge. Fistulous opening has hood of skin above the fistula (semilunar fold of skin with concavity downward as superior border of fistula). The opening moves up on deglutition and also with protrusion of the tongue.

Provisional Dignosis: Thyroglossal Fistula

Q.1 What is thyroglossal fistula?
Ans. It is acquired fistula which results either secondary to burst opened of infected thyroglossal cyst or following incomplete removal of thyroglossal cyst.

Causes are:
1. Secondary to incision and drainage of infected thyroglossal cyst.
2. Following burst opening of infected and abscess formed in thyroglossal cyst.
3. Following recurrence of incomplete removal.

Q.2 What is lining of fistula?

Ans. It is lined by columnar epithelium.

Q.3 What is "Hood sign"?

Ans. The skin above the fistulous opening is pulled upwards by the thyroglossal tract and this gives rise to puckering of the skin resembling a hood of a snake.

Q.4 What is the treatment?

Ans. Excision by transverse elliptical incision with excision of central part of hyoid bone with communicating duct.

Ranula

CASE: A tense spherical swelling in the floor of the mouth underneath, the tongue, in midline, measuring about 3 cm in diameter, blue tongue, smooth cystic and semitransparent.

Provisional Diagnosis: Ranula

Q.1 What is ranula?
Ans. It is a large mucous cyst in the floor of mouth of sublingual salivary gland or mucous gland of Blandin and Nuhn or more anteriorly placed gland of Suranne and Merkel near the incisor teeth. It present as a brilliantly translucent cystic swelling.

Q.2 Why is it called ranula?
Ans. Ranula resembles to the belly of a little frog hence the name ranula given by Hippocrates.

Q.3 What are the types of ranula?
Ans. Two types:
1. Simple ranula (oral).
2. Complex (deep or dissecting or plunging ranula or cervical ranula).

Q.4 Describe simple ranula?
Ans. It is relatively localized dilated segment of a blocked or damaged sublingual gland duct.

Q.5 What is plunging ranula?
Ans. Plunging is either an extension of simple ranula into the neck through the dehiscence into the mylohyoid muscle behind the submandibular gland or extravasated mucous escape (pseudocyst) from the posterior sublingual gland which burrow along the posterior margin of mylohyoid muscle down into the submandibular region and form a cervical swelling (Figs 1A and B).

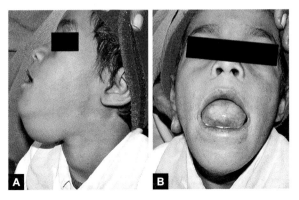

Figs 1A and B: Plunging ranula: (A) Submental swelling; (B) Swelling in floor of mouth

Q.6 What are features of simple ranula?

Ans. 1. It is a cystic swelling in the floor of the mouth under neath the tongue between symphysis menti and frenulum of the tongue.
2. Slow growing.
3. Just one side of the midline.
4. Spherical but one top part invisible.
5. Characteristic transparent gray appearance with blue tinge.
6. Smooth surface but the edge is difficult to feel.
7. Soft, fluctuant and transilluminates.
8. Noncompressible and nonreducible.
9. Cyst is not fixed.
10. It is tense, mucosa is stretched.
11. Wharton's ducts are seen runing over its surface.
12. Neck nodes: Not enlarged.
13. Frequent bursts and recurrence.

Q.7 What are dignostic features of plunging ranula?

Ans. Bidigital examination (one intraoral finger over the bulge and other in the neck). Plunging ranula presents as a acystic swelling in the floor of the tongue as well as in the sublingual/submental or submandibular region. It is bimanual palpable and inter linked.

Q.8 Describe pathology of ranula?

Ans. It has thin wall and composed of a delicate capsule of fibrous tissue. It is lined by columnar or cuboidal epithelium or fibrous tissue. It contains crystal clear, viscid and glairy or jelly-like fluid.

Q.9 What are complications?

Ans. Complications are:
1. Interference in mastication and swallowing.
2. Infection leading to Ludwig's angina.

    3. Ulceration.

    4. Interference in speech and articulation.

Q.10 What are differential diagnosis?

Ans. 1. Sublingual dermoid.

    2. Sebaceous cyst.

    3. Suprahyoid bursitis.

    4. Ludwig's angina.

    5. Lipoma.

    6. Lymphadenitis.

Q.11 How does a plunging ranula present clinically?

Ans. 1. First presents as oral swelling (45%).

    2. Oral and neck mass associated (34%).

    3. Only swelling in the neck (21%).

Q.12 What are the contents of plunging ranula?

Ans. High level of salivary amylase protein similar to secretion of sublingual gland.

Q.13 What is role of CT and MRI imaging?

Ans. Computed tomography scan and MRI can provide accurate localization of the mass. In CT and MR scan, a plunging ranula is characteristically cystic mass in the submandibular space that extends into or above the sublingual space (tail sign).

Q.14 What are various views for pathogenesis of plunging ranula?

Ans. Retension cyst of sublingual or submandibular gland that had gravitated into neck. Result of a mucous extravasation into the tissue from a traumatized sublingual gland or ducts. Its originates is from cervical sinus in a manner similar to that of a branchial cyst.

Q.15 What is pathogenesis of plunging ranula?

Ans. Plunging ranula is derived from extravasation of salivary secretion from sublingual gland and retension of saliva with extension into the neighbouring space. Parotid and submandibular gland secrete after major stimuli such as eating while sublingual secretes continuously during intradigestive period. Mucous extravasation occurs due to obstruction of salivary duct with resultant rupture of acini (due to increase in luminal pressure). Trauma, infection and anomalies of duct are prerequisites.

The pathway of mucous extravasation may be:

    1. Along the deep lobe of submandibular gland to exist posteriorly between hyoglossus and mylohyoid muscle.

    2. Directly through dehiscence of a hiatus in the mylohyoid muscle itself.

Q.16 What is treatment of simple ranula?

Ans. 1. Partial excision with marsupialization.

    2. Complete excision.

Q.17 What are treatment of plunging ranula?

Ans. 1. Intraoral excision by gental dissection leaving a drain from floor of the mouth down to the neck cavity.
   2. Cervical excision of cyst.
   3. Intraoral sublingual gland with drainage of cyst.
   4. Cervical excision with sublingual gland.

Q.18 What is marsupialization?

Ans. It consists of excision of roof along with overlying mucosa and apposition of cut edges of the mucous membrane of the floor of the mouth with cut edge of the remaining wall of mucosa. Thus, bottom of ranula forms the floor of mouth.

Occult Primary with Neck Node (Metastasis)

CASE: A patient present with a huge swelling left side of the neck of 9 months duration. It was painless increasing in size, hard and fixed to deeper structure (Fig. 1). No primary lesion could be detected in the thorough examination of the ear, nose and throat. Endoscopic examinations of the nose, nasopharynx, larynx and laryngopharynx were normal.

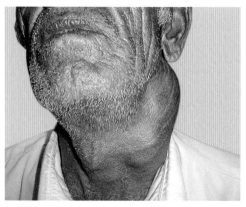

Fig. 1: Huge metastatic lymphadenopathy left side of neck

Provisional Diagnosis: Occult Primary with Neck Node

Q.1 What is the incidence of cervical metastasis?
Ans. 1. 80% of neck mass is cervical metastasis if thyroid is excluded.
    2. After 5th decades of life, about 90% of neck mass is malignant.

Q.2 What is the incidence of occult primary?
Ans. It is about 5% (3–9%).

Q.3 What is the treatment of metastasis lymph node with occult primary?
Ans. The treatment of metastasis lymph node with occult primary depends on:
    1. Level of lymph node, i.e. site.
    2. Size.
    3. Histology of lesion.

Q.4 What are the various sites of metastatic lymph nodes with occult primary?

Ans. These are as follows:
1. Preaccessory (infrastructure)—40%.
2. Mid-neck lateral jugulodigastric—(20%).
3. Lower cervical (10%).
4. Posterior-triangle accessory group (10%).
5. Others (10%).

Q.5 What are the various sites of primary in case of occult primary after therapy and during follow-up?

Ans. 1. Nasopharynx.
2. Base of tongue.
3. Pyriform fossa (apex).
4. Between anterior pillar and lingual attachment of tonsil.
5. Posterior pharyngeal wall.
6. Postcricoid.
7. Thyroid.
8. Subglottic.
9. Below the clavicle (esophagus, uterus, breast, testis).

Q.6 What investigations are usually done to locate occult primary?

Ans. 1. Triple endoscopy—repeated direct laryngoscopy, bronchoscopy and esophagoscopy.
2. Blind biopsy—successful in diagnosis only in 3–9% from fossa of Rosenmuller, base of the tongue and pyriform fossa.

Q.7 What are the various investigations to detect primary nasopharynx?

Ans. 1. Postnasal mirror examination
2. Yaunkauer speculum examination.
3. Endoscopic examination of nasopharynx.
4. Flexible nasopharyngoscopy.
5. Blind biopsy.
6. Contrast study.
7. CT scan and MRI.

Q.8 What are the various investigations to detect primary in subglottic region?

Ans. 1. Mirror examination (I/L).
2. Direct laryngoscopy with or without mirror.
3. Subglotticoscope.
4. Retrograde bronchoscopy.
5. Transconioscope.
6. Flexible bronchoscopy.
7. Contrast study.
8. CT scan.
9. MRI.
10. Open laryngofissure.

Q.9 What should be the approach for patient with occult primary?

Ans. Approach should be:

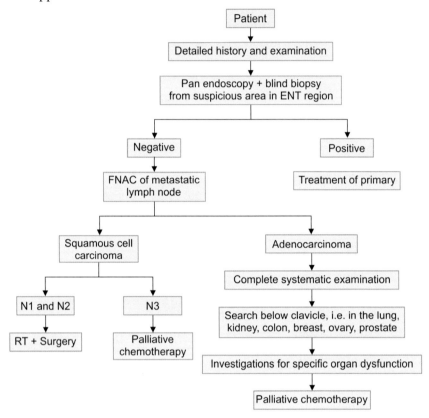

Submandibular Sialadenitis

CASE: A swelling in the submandibular region which increases during meals and becomes painful. The swelling is palpable on bimanual digital examination. It is ovoid (almond shaped), firm and has smooth lobulated surface (Fig. 1).

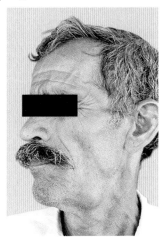

Fig. 1: Submandibular swelling (sialadenitis)

Provisional Diagnosis: Submandibular Sialadenitis

Q.1 What are points in favor of diagnosis?

Ans. Points are:
1. The gland is swollen.
2. Swelling increases during and after meals.
3. Swelling becomes painful during and after meals and becomes tense and tender.
4. It is palpable on bidigital examination.
5. With lemon juice saliva flows freely from the nonaffected side while it is absent or scanty on affected side.
6. Stone may be palpable in the duct on bimanual digital examination.
7. Overlying skin: Normal and freely mobile.

Q.2 Why is submandibular gland palpable on bidigital examination?

Ans. Deep lobe of submandibular salivary gland is deep to myelohyoid muscle, so when the gland is enlarged, it is palpable on bidigital examination. Lymph node is superficial to myelohyoid, so not palpable.

Q.3 What are other clinical findings in submandibular sialoadenitis?

Ans. These are:

1. Asymmetrical floor of the mouth.
2. The orifice of duct in the floor of the mouth is red and edematous on affected side.
3. There may be pus or watery or mucopurulent discharge from duct opening (due to partial obstruction) on pressing the gland on bidigital palpation.

Q.4 What is salivary calculus?

Ans. Salivary stone is formed by cellular debris and mucous mixed with phosphates and carbonates of calcium and magnesium.

Q.5 Why stone formation is common in submandibular salivary gland?

Ans. 80% stones are formed in submandibular gland. Several causes are:

1. High mucin contents of secretion which is more viscus.
2. Secretion is rich in salts.
3. Secretion flow is against gravity.
4. Terminal opening end of the duct is narrow like bottle neck while that of the parotid is like flask.
5. The floor of the mouth is site for stagnation of saliva, contamination and infection where the duct opens.
6. Duct pursues long and curved course.
7. The more acidic PH of the secretion.
8. More chances of affection of its parasympathetic nerve fibers (corda tympani nerve) causing secretomotor dysfunction and thus impairing flow of the saliva.

Q. 6 How will you proceed for confirmation of diagnosis?

Ans. 1. By-clinical examination.
2. X-ray: Lateral oblique view of submandibular region for stone in the gland.
3. Occlusal view (X-ray) floor of the mouth for stone in the Wharton's duct.
(If mineral content is 30% or more, opaque shadow is visible).

Q.7 What is importance of X-ray of occlusal view of floor of the mouth in salivary calculus?

Ans. It will show the calculi in the hilum of the gland and extraglandular duct system.

Q.8 What is the differential diagnosis of a radiopaque shadow in X-ray of occlusal view of floor of the mouth?

Ans. A shadow of stone can mimic with calcified lymph node or phlebolith.

Q.9 In which condition the submandibular salivary stone is not visualized in X-ray?

Ans. 1. In Wharton's duct in the region of right angle bend (coma area) around the posterior border of mylohyoid muscle.

2. Inaccurate positioning of film so the lingual balcony of projecting mandibular cortical bone.

3. Superimposition of mandible.

Q.10 What are common sites of stone formation in salivary gland?

Ans. 1. At the anterior border of masseter muscle in parotid.

2. At the posterior border of mylohyoid in submandibular gland.

Q.11 Which muscles are supplied by ramus mandibularis?

Ans. 1. Depressor angularis and orbicularis oris.

2. Other muscles of lips.

3. Muscles of chin.

Q.12 What is the % of radiolucens of salivary gland stone?

Ans. It is 20%.

Q.13 What are common differential diagnosis?

Ans. These are:

1. Enlarged lymph node.

2. Lateral ranula.

3. Lateral sublingual cervical dermoid.

4. Lipoma.

5. Neurofibroma.

Q.14 What is treatment?

Ans. Treatment depends on the site and size of stone.

1. If the stone is larger and is in main duct: It is removed by making a longitudinal incision over the stone under local anesthesia. The wound is not sutured. If a stricture is formed at the site of incision, the duct is repaired with a procedure sialodochoplasty. If recurrence occur, gland is removed.

2. If stone is small in size but in the duct little bit posterior, it is removed under GA.

3. If stone is in the gland or very far part of the duct, or if there is recurrence: Excision of gland.

Q.15 What important structures are liable to be injured during operation?

Ans. 1. Marginal mandibular branch of facial nerve (ramus mandibularis) (If injured, patient is unable to pucker his lips normally).

2. Lingual nerve.

3. Hypoglossal nerve.

4. Facial artery and vein.

Q.16 What are the causes of recurrences of salivary duct stone?

Ans. Causes are:

1. Continuation of basic inflammation.
2. Residual fibrous stricture.
3. Irregular duct wall.

Q.17 What are indications of submandibular salivary gland excision?

Ans. 1. Chronic submandibular sialoadenitis.
2. Stone in gland or its hilum.
3. Recurrence salivary gland duct stone.
4. Submandibular salivary fistula.
5. Stricture of Wharton's duct.
6. As a part of radical neck dissection.
7. Traumatic injury of gland: Unrepairable.
8. Benign tumor of gland.
9. Malignant tumor of salivary gland.
10. Tuberculosis of salivary gland.
11. Sarcoidosis.

Mixed Parotid Tumor (Pleomorphic Salivary Gland Tumor)

CASE: Slow-growing painless swelling in the parotid region (Fig. 1), of about 5 cm in diameter, firm, lobulated surface. The swelling is not adherent to the masseter muscle. Overlying skin is free. Facial nerve is normal. Ear lobule is raised. No regional lymph node is enlarged.

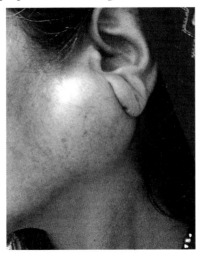

Fig. 1: Parotid swelling

Provisional Diagnosis: Mixed Parotid Tumor

Q.1 What are the points in favor of parotid swelling?
Ans. It is a parotid swelling because:
1. Swelling is below, in front and behind the ear lobule obliterating the normal furrow behind the ramus of the mandible.
2. The lobule of the ear is lifted up.

Q.2 What are the points in favor of mixed parotid tumor?
Ans. The points in favor are:
1. It is in the parotid region.
2. Swelling is painless, slow growing and lobulated.

3. It is mobile, skin is not fixed.
4. Facial nerve is not involved.
5. Regional lymph nodes are not involved.

Q.3 What is parotid region?

Ans. It is a region which is more or less bounded.
   1. Above: By zygoma.
   2. Below: By line joining angle of mouth to mastoid process.
   3. Anteriorly: By anterior border of masseter muscle.
   4. Posteriorly: By mastoid process.

Q.4 What is the significance of parotid region?

Ans. Lump in this region is considered a swelling of the parotid gland origin until proved otherwise.

Q.5 How a parotid swelling is examined?

Ans. Parotid is examined by Mnemonic "PAROTIDS":
   P—Parotid region.
   A—auricle or adjoining region.
   R—regional area or relation with skin, muscle or bone.
   O—obliteration of retromandibular sulcus or orbit examination or ocular.
   T—temporomandibular joint.
   I—intraoral examination (deep lobe and duct's opening).
   D—ducts (Stensen's duct).
   S—seventh nerve (facial nerve).

Q.6 Which is the most common tumor of parotid gland?

Ans. 1. Benign tumors are 80%
   2. Malignant tumors are 20%
   3. Pleomorphic adenoma (mixed tumor) is the most common benign tumor.
   4. Mucoepidermoid tumor is the most common malignant tumor.

Q.7 Why a pleomorphic adenoma is called mixed tumor?

Ans. There are different type of cells in the tumor. Actually, they derive from columnar or squamous epithelial cell by mucoid degeneration. The epithelial cells shows various forms, so it is called pleomorphic adenoma.

Q.8 Is it truly benign?

Ans. It is benign but potentially malignant.
   1. Capsule is deficient
   2. Recurrence is common after excision
   3. May undergo malignant change (about 2.5%).

Q.9 What are the points that suggest its malignant conversion?

Ans. If it changes and shows the following:
   1. Sudden rapid growth in long-standing tumor.
   2. Sudden pain.

3. Becoming fix to skin, muscle or bone.
4. Presence of facial nerve palsy.
5. Enlargment of cervical lymph nodes.
6. Restricted jaw movements.
7. Infiltration of surrounding tissue.
8. Hard and irregular mass.

Q.10 How does salivary gland tumor classified?

Ans. International classification of salivary gland tumors is as follows:

I. Epithelial tumor:
   A. Adenoma:
      1. Monomorphic, e.g. adenolymphoma, oxyphilic adenoma, others.
      2. Pleomorphic.
   B. Mucoepidermoid tumor
   C. Acinic cell tumor
   D. Carcinomas:
      1. Carcinoma in pleomorphic adenoma
      2. Adenoid cystic carcinoma
      3. Adenocarcinoma
      4. Epidermoid
      5. Anaplastic.

II. Nonepithelial tumor (Rare)
   A. (1) Benign hemangioma; (2) Lipoma; (3) Neurofibroma
   B. Malignant: (1) Rhabdomyosarcoma; (2) Liposarcoma.

Q.11 What are the probable causes of swelling in the parotid region?

Ans. 1. Neoplastic (75%).
   2. Non-neoplastic:
      a. Acute and chronic parotitis.
      b. Parotid calculi.
      c. Acute unilateral or bilateral (mumps).
      d. Malformation: Lymphangioma, hemangioma,
      e. Cysts.
      f. Chronic infection: tuberculosis, sarcoidosis.
   3. Miscellaneous causes:
      a. Drugs: Antithyroid, iodides, antidepressant.
      b. Sialosis enlargement due to metabolic or hormonal, diabetes, acromegaly.
      c. Mikulicz and Sjogren's disease and syndromes.

Q.12 How will you confirm your diagnosis in parotid mixed tumor?

Ans. 1. Clinical ground.
   2. FNAC.
   3. Sonography.
   4. MRI and CT scan.

Q.13 What are the new investigations for salivary disease?

Ans. 1. Diagnostic sialendoscopy.

2. Therapeutic sailendoscopy procedures for removal of debris, dilatation of stricture.

Q.14 What is the differential diagnosis?

Ans. These are:

1. Lipoma: It is soft-lobulated, margin slips under the examining finger.
2. Neurofibroma: It is usually fusiform, firm to rubbery in consistency, often multiple. It may be tender.
3. Sebaceous cyst: It is cystic, adherent skin, punctum is present.
4. Bony tumor: Bony hard and attached to bone.
5. Preauricular lymph node: Firm smooth swelling just in front of tragus, usually mobile and outside of the parotid capsule.
6. Warthin's tumor: It is usually in tail of parotid gland, more common in male, tumor is soft, smooth surface and often fluctuates.

Q.15 What is sialography?

Ans. 1. It is contrast radiological study to visualize the ductal system of salivary gland.

2. A watery solution of lipoidal is injected into the orifice of Stensen's duct (open in the buccal surface of the cheek opposite the upper second molar tooth).
3. It will demonstrate:
   i. Any obstruction of the duct
   ii. Dilatation of the duct and acini (sialectasis)
   iii. Locate the site of lesion in parotid fistula.

Q.16 What are the complications of pleomorphic salivary adenoma?

Ans. 1. Malignant transformation.

2. Recurrence (often multicentric).

Q.17 What are peculiarities of mixed tumor in gross pathology?

Ans. 1. It arises from acini of the parotid, unicentric or may be multicentric.

2. Capsule is thin and composed of compression of the surrounding salivary tissue.
3. Capsule is incomplete, nodular or small tissue of the tumor project out through the defects in the normal salivary tissue.
4. It is variable in size from a plum to fetal head.

Q.18 What is the treatment of mixed tumor?

Ans. Superficial parotidectomy: Facial nerve is preserved. If deep lobe is involved, total parotidectomy is done.

Q.19 What precautions will be taken for the operation of superficial parotidectomy?

Ans. Proper consent and information of patient and asking his relatives regarding the possibilities of the followings:

1. Chances of facial paresis or paralysis.

    2. Chances of Frey's syndrome.

    3. Recurrences.

Q.20 What are the causes of recurrence following operation on mixed parotid tumor?

Ans. 1. Incomplete pseudocapsule.

    2. Inadequate and incomplete removal.

    3. Implantation—recurrence during manipulation by spilage, dominate biological behavior.

    4. Multicentric origin of tumor.

Malignant Tumor of Parotid Gland

CASE: A stony-hard swelling at parotid region which is fixed to the muscle and bone. Skin is fixed and ulcerated (Fig. 1). Facial nerve paralysis is present. Cervical lymph node is enlarged and palpable.

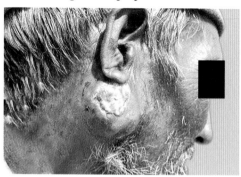

Fig. 1: Parotid swelling with ulceration over it

Provisional Diagnosis: Malignant Tumor of Parotid Gland

Q.1 What are the points in favor of facial nerve palsy?
Ans. 1. Loss of nasolabial fold.
    2. Drooping of angle of mouth.
    3. Widening of palpebral fissure.
    4. Drooping of lower eye lid with epiphora.
    5. Loss of wrinkling of forehead.
    6. On active movement and procedure:
        a. Failure to close the affected side eye.
        b. Failure to elevate eyebrow on affected side.
        c. Failure to blow out (air leaks on affected side).
        d. On asking to show teeth, angle of mouth deviate to normal side.

Q.2 What are the peculiarities of parotid malignant tumor?
Ans. 1. Low-grade malignant tumor (like mucoepidermoid or acinic cell tumor) does not involve the facial nerve at an early stage like benign, so it is difficult to clinically diagnose.

    2. Adenocarcinoma and anaplastic carcinoma involve the facial nerve in early stage.

    3. Adenoid cystic carcinoma has strong tendency to involve the nerve and to spread along perineural sheath.

Q.3 How is diagnosis confirmed?
Ans. 1. If parotid swelling is mobile and no facial palsy by FNAC.

    2. If parotid swelling is fixed with facial palsy tumor by open biopsy.

Q.4 What are slow-growing malignancy tumor?
Ans. Slow-growing tumors are mucoepidermoid, acinic cell tumors and adenoid cystic carcinoma.

Q.5 What are rapidly growing malignancies?
Ans. These are adenocarcinoma, anaplastic carcinoma and 25% of mucoepidermoid carcinoma.

Q.6 What is the treatment of malignant parotid tumors?
Ans. 1. Total parotidectomy with facial nerve preservation in mucoepidermoid carcinoma and acinic cell carcinoma without facial palsy.

    2. Total parotidectomy (nerve may be grafted with great auricular nerve) in hard tumor with facial nerve palsy.

    3. Radical excision including mandible and muscle in hard and fixed tumor.

    4. Radical excision with block dissection neck in tumor with cervical lymph node metastasis.

    5. Palliative radiotherapy for inoperable tumor.

SECTION 3

Diseases of Throat (Oral Cavity, Pharynx and Larynx)

- Carcinoma Lip
- Leukoplakia
- Epulis
- Carcinoma of the Tongue
- Oral Cancer
- Oral Submucous Fibrosis
- Chronic Tonsillitis
- Enlarged Adenoids
- Vocal Cord Nodules (Singer's Nodule)
- Vocal Cord Polyp
- Contact Ulcer Larynx
- Unilateral Vocal Cord Paralysis
- Juvenile Multiple Papilloma Larynx
- Cancer Larynx
- Malignancy Pyriform Fossa
- Postcricoid Carcinoma

CASE

33 Carcinoma Lip

CASE: Painless ulcer on the upper or lower lip and angle of mouth (Fig. 1) which does not heal even with medical treatment. It bleeds on touch, submental lymph node may be enlarged.

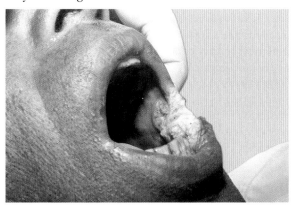

Fig. 1: Ulcerative growth angle of lip and lateral part

Provisional Diagnosis: Carcinoma Lip

Q.1 Why is it carcinomatous ulcer?

Ans. Points in favor are:
1. Initial lesion started as a small nodule, which ultimately ulcerated.
2. Fixed to underlying tissue.
3. Edges are everted and raised.
4. Blood-stained discharge.
5. A hard and discrete submental lymph node.

Q.2 What are predisposing factors?

Ans. Predisposing factors are:
1. Age common between 60 and 70 years.
2. Predominantly in male.
3. Common in lower lip (93%) because of exposure to sunlight and tobacco chewing.

4. Commonly in farmers (exposed to ultraviolet rays).
5. Common in people who has actinic cheilitis due to prolonged exposure to sunlight (repeated cracking and desquamation to form erosion of lip).
6. Speckled leukoplakia.
7. Khaini: Keeping between lower lip and gum.

Q.3 What are the various sites?
Ans. The various sites are: lower lip (93%), upper lip (5%), angle of mouth (2%).

Q.4 Which site is more malignant among various sites of carcinomatous lesion of the lip?
Ans. Carcinoma at the angle of the mouth is more malignant because the angle has double lymphatic drainage.

Q.5 What are the clinical appearances of lip carcinoma?
Ans. Lip carcinoma is either nodular or ulcerative.
1. Nodular: It is due to proliferative type, cauliflower like or warty growth or thickned indurated mass.
2. Ulcerative type: It is persistent painless ulceration (refuses to heal) often with bleeding, offensive discharge or crust formation. Nontender with thin watery.
3. The area around the growth may show blistering, thickening pigmentation or white boggy patches.
4. Base is indurated, advanced lesion is fixed to gum and jaw; metastatic lymph nodes are hard, discrete and nontender.

Q.6 What is lymphatic drainage of lip?
Ans. 1. The lymphatic from the center of lower lip drains into submental lymph node then to lower deep cervical lymph node.
2. Lymphatic from side of lower lip drains to middle cervical lymph node.
3. Lymphatic from upper lip passes across the face and over the angle of the mandible to upper deep cervical lymph nodes.
4. Lymphatic from the angle of the mouth drains into the lymphatic of both lips.

Q.7 What is the differential diagnosis?
Ans. Many conditions like:
1. Chancre of the lip
2. Molluscum-sebaceum (Keratoacanthoma)
3. Ectopic salivary tumor
4. Herpetic ulcer
5. Traumatic ulcer
6. Hemangioma
7. Papilioma
8. Neurofibroma.

Q.8 How is diagnosis confirmed?
Ans. By biopsy which shows squamous cell carcinoma.

Q.9 What are the other investigations to be done?

Ans. 1. Blood for VDRL to exclude syphilis.
   2. X-ray of the chest.
   3. X-ray of the jaw.
   4. Routine blood test.

Q.10 What is the line of treatment?

Ans. 1. Radiotherapy: Treatment of choice, if lesion is less than 2 cm in diameter.
   2. Surgery: Indicated in:
      a. Carcinoma supervening leukoplakia or syphilitic sores
      b. Failed radiotherapy
      c. Late cases: Lesion more than 2 cm
      d. Involvement of jaw.
   3. Chemotherapy: Radiotherapy may be combined with chemotherapy for advanced cases.

Q.11 What is the treatment of metastatic cervical lymph node?

Ans. 1. Regional lymph node are mobile—classical block dissection.
   2. Regional lymph nodes are fixed—palliative radiotherapy.

CASE

34

Leukoplakia

CASE: White opaque rough patch with irregular wrinkles and varying degrees of induration at places, on the cheek mucosa.

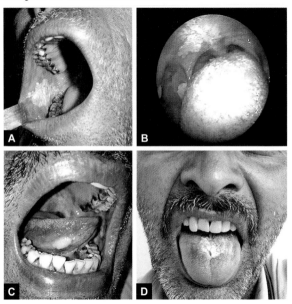

Figs 1A to D: (A) Leukoplakia of the buccal mucosa; (B) Leukoplakia of the palate;
(C) Hypertrophic leukoplakia of the tongue; (D) Leukoplakia on the surface of tongue

Provisional Diagnosis: Leukoplakia

Q.1 What is leukoplakia?
Ans. Leukoplakia (Leuko=White, Plak= Plaque) is a white moist hyperkeratotic patch commonly occurring in the mouth (Figs 1A and B), tongue (Figs 1C and D), larynx, and some other mucosa in response to irritation.

Q.2 What are the predisposing factors?
Ans. Chronic and persistent irritation by:
1. Spirit.
2. Smoking.

3. Spices (betel nut, tobacco, pan, etc.).
4. Syphilis.
5. Sepsis (including candidiasis).
6. Sharp ragged tooth.
7. Susceptibility.

Q.3 What is the characteristic nature of leukoplakia?
Ans. It is premalignant lesion, particularly, speckled leukoplakia.

Q.4 What is the differential diagnosis?
Ans. White patches are produced by:
1. Lichen planus (striated fine lace-like patches, has self-limiting course and response with local application of glucocorticoids.
2. Nicotine induced stomatitis.
3. Hyperkeratosis due to friction.
4. Avitaminosis.
5. Candidiasis infection.

Q.5 What are the types of leukoplakia?
Ans. Leukoplakia may be:
1. Simple (Homogeneous): Patches or flacks or soft white velvety areas on the mucosa without palpable induration.
2. Complex: Many forms can occur:
   a. Verrucous leukoplakia (nodular): Speckled warty surfaces and varying degree of induration.
   b. Leukoerythroplakia (erosive) red-colored with vascular leukoplakia and extremely malignant potential.

Q.6 What is the relation of pathological and clinical features in leukoplakia?
Ans. 1. Stage I (Hyperkeratosis): Clinically milky, bluish, thin gray transparent film on mucosa.
2. Stage II (Acanthosis or hyperplasia): Clinically smooth, thick, opaque white paint like enamel of tooth.
3. Stage III (Dyskeratosis): Clinically shiny red, dry rough white patch, scattered raw beef appearance with cracks or irregular wrinkles.
4. Stage IV (Carcinoma in situ): Clinically manifests as fissures or warty projections or small nodular or raw glazed area in middle of white area (erythropakia) with induration.

Q.7 What is the chance of malignant transformation in leukoplakia?
Ans. It varies from 1 to 17%, average about 5% become malignant.

Q.8 What is the treatment of leukoplakia?
Ans. 1. Avoid the identified irritations.
2. Treatment of associated candidiasis: Local treatment with nystatin fluconazole.
3. Excision—(a) Surgical: (b) Laser; (c) Cobalation.
4. Close follow-up.

CASE: A pinkish nodule arising from the lateral surface of the gum at premolar tooth region left upper side, which is firm, nontender and pedunculated (Fig. 1).

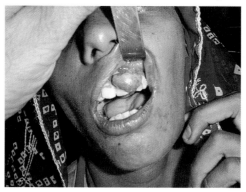

Fig. 1: Nodular swelling of the gum at left upper premolar region

Provisional Diagnosis: Epulis

Q.1 What is epulis?

Ans. Epulis means "upon the gum", any swelling on the gum is epulis. Actually it is localized enlargement of gum.

Q.2 What are the points in favor of diagnosis?

Ans. These are:
1. Pink nodule arising from gum.
2. Nodule is firm, nontender.
3. Slow-growing mass.
4. Nonfriable and does not bleed on touch.
5. Usually at the site of premolar tooth which is loose.
6. Draining lymph node is not enlarged.

Q.3 What are the different types of epulis?

Ans. The different types of epulis are:
1. Fibrous
2. Myeloid

3. Granulomatous
4. Carcinomatous

Q.4 What are the features of fibrous epulis?
Ans. It is firm, pinkish in color, nodular, nontender swelling arising from the gum and does not bleed on touch.

Q.5 What are the features of granulomatous epulis?
Ans. It is soft-red swelling which bleeds on touch and is related to caries tooth.

Q.6 What are the features of myeloid epulis?
Ans. It is firm, purple-colored rapidly growing mass.

Q.7 What are the features of carcinomatous type of epulis?
Ans. It is actually fungating growth. The mass may be painfull friable and has bleeding tendency. Regional lymph nodes are enlarged.

Q.8 What is the differential diagnosis of epulis?
Ans. Odontogenic tumors and actinomycosis.

Q.9 What are the pathological features of fibrous epulis?
Ans. The pathological features are as follows:
1. It is the most common variety.
2. Arises from periodontal membrane at the neck of the incisor or premolar teeth.
3. Pathologically it arises from interdental papilla or in response to local irritation (from sharp margin of carious cavity).
4. More common in women.
5. Common in young adults (about 30 years of age).

Q.10 What are the salient clinical features of fibrous epulis?
Ans. 1. It is slow growing.
2. About 1–3 cm in size.
3. Polypoidal in shape.
4. Usually round or ovoid but may resemble thick flat disc.
5. Firm in consistency.
6. Pedunculated but pedicle may be too short, so it appears, to be sessile.
7. Smooth surface with normal gingival color.
8. The adjacent teeth are irregularly displaced.
9. Lymph nodes are not enlarged.

Q.11 What is the treatment of epulis?
Ans. Excision of epulis with cautry of the base to stop bleeding.

Carcinoma of the Tongue

CASE: Ulcerative growth with rolled out and everted edge; indurated base and slough in floor in the center on the lateral side of the tongue (Figs 1A and B).

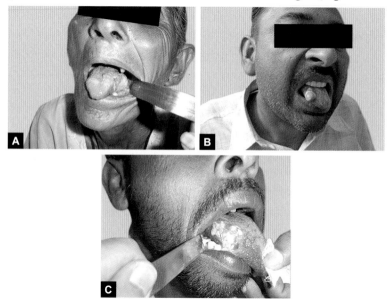

Figs 1A to C: Different site showing ulcerative growth of the tongue

Provisional Diagnosis: Carcinoma of the Tongue

Q.1 What are the predisposing factors of cancer tongue?
Ans. These are:
1. 6 S—smoking, spirit (alcohol), spices (betel nut, betel leaf, gutaka, etc.), sepsis (including candidiasis), sharp ragged teeth and syphilis.
2. Avitaminosis
3. Plummer Vinsen's syndrome

4. Oral submucous fibrosis
5. Papilloma
6. Fissured tongue
7. Superficial atrophic glossitis.

Q.2 What are its premalignant conditions?
Ans. These are leukoplakia (warty or verrucous type), erythroplakia, melanoplakia, and oral submucous fibrosis, papilloma.

Q.3 What are the various sites of the tongue for cancer?
Ans 1. Dorsum of the tongue (90%)
    – Lateral border at middle one-third of tongue (50%)
    – Posterior one-third tongue (20%)
    – Tip of the tongue (10%)
  2. Dorsum toward the midline (10%)
    – Under surface of the tongue (10%).

Q.4 What are the common gross pathological presentations of growth?
Ans. The microscopic appearances are:
1. Proliferative: (cauliflower or exophytic) or warty nodule (Fig. 1C).
2. Ulcerative: With rolled out and everted edge.
3. Cracks or fissures: With induration all-round.
4. Diffuse type: Indurated tongue with early fixity (frozen tongue) but without any visible lesion.
5. Indurated plaque: Submucous nodule.

Q.5 How does local spread of cancer tongue occur?
Ans. Local spread occurs by infiltration and implantation to adjacent areas depending on site of origin.
1. Anterior two-third tongue growth spreads to the floor of mouth.
2. Junction of anterior two-third and posterior one-third to mandible.
3. Posterior one-third of tongue: Growth spreads to different direction:
    a. Laterally to involve the tonsil and lateral pharyngeal wall
    b. Posteriorly into epiglottis
    c. Downward into the larynx
    d. Medially to opposite side
    e. Temporomandibular joint.

Q.6 What are the peculiarities of lymphatic spread in cancer tongue?
Ans. Early metastasis deposition in the lymph node occurs because of the following reasons:
1. Tongue is rich in lymphatic.
2. Criss-cross interlacing muscle fibres of the tongue muscles.
3. Constant movement of the tongue, both produce or squeezing of lymphatic and help in early dissemination in the lymphatic by embolic spread.

Q.7 What are the various sites for lymph node metastasis?

Ans. 1. From lip to submental or submandibular then to either or both jugulo-omohyid lymph node.

2. From anterior one-third tongue to submandibular and then jugulo-omohyoid (same side).

3. In late stage when growth cross the midline, metastasis can occur to opposite side lymph node.

4. From posterior one-third tongue to jugulodigastric lymph node (both side). The lymphatic from the tongue passes from the floor of the mouth to the regional lymph node through the periosteum of the mandible not through the mandible itself.

Q.8 Can the cancer spread by hematogenous route?

Ans. Not an early feature but growth of posterior third tongue may give secondaries in the lung.

Q.9 What are the common symptoms of cancer tongue?

Ans. 1. Pre-existing history of either leukoplakia or predisposing factor may be present.

2. Painless lump, ulcer or irregularity on the tongue commonly at lateral side.

3. Excessive salivation (stimulation of parotid gland).

4. Referred pain in the ear (irritation of lingual nerve to auricular temporal nerve).

5. Halitosis.

6. Ankyloglossia.

7. Defective articulation.

8. Trismus.

9. Pain (due to infiltration and involvement of lingual nerve).

Q.10 What is fate or terminal events in cancer tongue?

Ans. 1. Hemorrhage: Due to erosion of lingual artery or internal carotid artery in posterior third tongue.

2. Cachexia and starvation.

3. Aspiration pneumonia.

4. Asphyxia (edma larynx or presser by metastatic gland on air passage).

Q.11 What are the treatment modalities of cancer tongue?

Ans. 1. For primary lesion:

Radiotherapy indications are:

– Lesion less than 2 cm in all diameter.

– Lesion of posterior one-third tongue.

– Inoperable cases of anterior two-third tongue.

2. Surgery indications are:

– Small tumor close to lip.

– Small tumor on dorsum.

– Carcinoma in preexisting precarcinoma lesion.

– Recurrence following radiotherapy.

– Lesion involving mandible.

3. Treatment for metastatic lymph node:
   - Radical neck dissection: Mobile nodes persisting for 3 weeks.
4. Mobile nodes metastesis present.
   - Palliative radiotherapy: In significant and fixed nodes.

Q.12 What are the common surgical procedures?

Ans. 1. Wedge resection: In case of tip of tongue.
2. Partial or oblique glossectomy: Lateral border of anterior one-third tongue.
3. Hemiglossectomy: lateral border of anterior two-thirds tongue.
4. Total glossectomy:
   a. Diffuse carcinoma;
   b. Recurrent cancer.
5. Commando (hemiglossectomy, excision of adjacent floor of mouth and mandible with RND) on side with floor of the mouth with 2 cm of jaw.

Oral Cancer

CASE: A rapidly spreading nonhealing ulcer with indurated base and everted edge, friable on the cheek mucosa. Regional cervical lymph node enlarged and palpable.

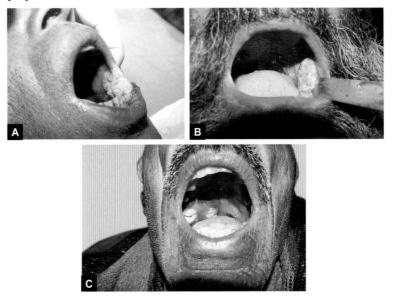

Figs 1A to C: Showing different site of oral cancer

Provisional Diagnosis: Oral Cancer

Q.1 What are the common sites of oral cancer?
Ans. Common sites are:
1. Buccal mucosa (more in cheek) (Figs 1A and B)
2. Lower alveolus
3. Lower sulcus
4. Floor of the mouth
5. Tongue
6. Palate (Fig. 1C)
7. Lip.

Q.2 What are predisposing or precancerous factors in oral cancer?

Ans. 1. Chewing tobacco and betel (pan) in cheek cancer and sucking tobacco bolus (khaini) in gingival cancer.
2. Smoking bidies or reverse bidi (hard palatal cancer).
3. Chronic irritation from ill-fitting denture, sharp jagged teeth.
4. Smoking of clay pipe (lip cancer).
5. Chronic superficial glossitis.
6. Leukoplakia specially candida infected speckled leukoplakia and erythroplakia (more in cheek mucosa).
7. Alcohol.
8. Papilloma.
9. Oral submucous fibrosis.

Q.3 What are the different gross appearances?

Ans. 1. Exophytic: Cauliflower like growth.
2. Infiltrating ulcer: Spreading deeply into the adjoining underlying tissue.

Q.4 How does the oral cancer spread?

Ans. 1. Direct extensions: To involve the mandible, alveolus, maxilla, skin of cheek, infratemporal fossa and pterygoid muscle (trismus).
2. Lymphatic: To regional nodes, upper cervical nodes.
3. Hematogenous: Rare to lungs, liver, bone, etc.

Q.5 What are the complications or terminal features of oral cancer?

Ans. The complications of oral cancer are:
1. Bronchopneumonia
2. Uncontrolled hemorrhage
3. Cachexia.

Q.6 What is the differential diagnosis?

Ans. 1. Traumatic ulcer.
2. Tubercular ulcer.
3. Dyspeptic ulcer.

Q.7 What investigations are required in oral cancer?

Ans. 1. X-ray mandible or maxilla to assess spread into bone.
2. X-ray chest PA view.
3. Biopsy.

Q.8 What are the stages for oral cancer?

Ans. 1. Stage I—T1 N0 M0
2. Stage II—T2 N0 M0
3. Stage III—T3 N0 M0 or T3 N1 M0
4. Stage IV—T4 N0 or N1 M0, Any TN2 or N3 or any N M1.

Q.9 What is meant by TNM classification?

Ans.

Tx— Inadequate information to assess the tumor.

T0— No evidence of tumor.

T1— Greater diameter less than 2 cm.
T2— Greater diameter between 2 and 4 cm.
T3— Greater diameter more than 4 cm.
T4— More than 4 cm with deep invasion (muscle/bone).
NX— Inadequate information to assess nodes.
N0— No clinically evidence of nodes.
N1— Single clinically positive homolateral node between 3 and 6 cm.
N2— Multiple homolateral nodes less than 6 cm.
N3— Massive homolateral, bilateral or contralateral nodes.
MX— Inadequate information to assess metastasis.
M0— No evidence of distant metastasis.
M1— Distant metastasis present.

Q.10 What is the treatment?
Ans. Treatment comprises of:
1. Treatment of primary:
   T1 and T2—by surgery or by irradiation
   Surgery: It is indicated in:
   a. T1 and T2
   b. Recurrence following RT
   c. Tumor involving bone
   d. Bulky tumor
   e. Cancer over preexisting leukoplakia
   Radiotherapy: By radium mould, radium, cobalt beam
   Chemotherapy: As an adjustment or palliation treatment of secondary
2. Treatment for secondary nodes (Metastasis)
   Block dissection: Mobile lymph nodes
   Radiotherapy for fixed metastasis nodes.

Oral Submucous Fibrosis

CASE: A patient presents with progressive restricted opening of the mouth with history of burning pain on taking chilies and spicy food for last 3 years. He is habitual of chewing betel nut and gutaka for last 4 years. On examination of the oral cavity there is blanching, fibrosis and increased hardness of mucosa of the soft palate, buccal mucosa. Uvula is reverted (Figs 1A and B).

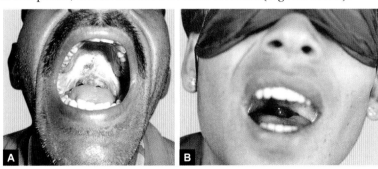

Figs 1A and B: (A) Oral submucous fibrosis (SMF); (B) Oral SMF with trismus

Provisional Diagnosis: Oral Submucous Fibrosis

Q.1 What is submucous fibrosis (SMF)?
Ans. It is chronic insidious disease of the oral cavity characterized by juxtra-epithelial deposition of fibrous tissue in the oral cavity and sometimes in the pharynx.

Q.2 What is historical background of SMF?
Ans. The disease was first described in India by Joshi in 1953. Desa described the condition in detail with sequence of events and hence, it also bears his name "Desa syndrome".

Q.3 What are the etiological factors associated with oral SMF?
Ans. The disease is common in Indian subcontinent. The prevalence rate varies from 2 to 5 per 1000.

Exact etiology is not known. Several factors claimed are:
1. Prolonged local irritation:
   a. Chewing betel nut alone or with betel leaf—causes mechanical irritation by rough surface or by chemical arecoline.
   b. Chewing of tobacco or smoking.
   c. Excessive chilies and spicy food.
2. Dietary deficiency: Vitamin B complex and vitamin A and iron deficiency.
3. Localized collagen disease: Histological changes are similar to those found in other collagen disease, e.g. rheumatoid arthritis, scleroderma.
4. Racial: More common in Indian or people of Indian origin living abroad.

Q.4 What are histological features of oral SMF?
Ans. 1. Fibrosis in lamina propria.
   2. Atrophy of the epithelium.
   3. Exposure of nerve ending.
   4. Later on fibrosis becomes marked causing progressive trismus and ankyloglossia.
   5. It is considered as premalignant condition, associated leukoplakia, malignant transformation can occur in 3–7.6% of cases.

Q.5 What are common symptoms of SMF?
Ans. 1. Soreness in mouth.
   2. Burning sensation increase on taking chilies or spicy food.
   3. Vesicular eruption and ulceration on the palate.
   4. Reduced mouth opening
   5. Deficiency in protruding the tongue.

Q.6 What are common sites involved in oral SMF?
Ans. The common sites of fibrosis are:
   1. Soft palate.
   2. Faucial pillars.
   3. Buccal mucosa.

Q.7 What is the treatment of oral SMF?
Ans. 1. Avoid irritant like betel nuts, pan, tobacco and spicy food.
   2. Treatment of anemia and vitamin A and vitamin B complex deficiency.
   3. Topical injection of steroid.
   4. Topical steroid and hylase injection.
   5. Oral steroid.

Q.8 What are various surgical treatment of oral SMF?
Ans. 1. Laser beam (CO_2) cutting the fibrous bands.
   2. Excision of fibrous bands and skin grafting.
   3. Excision of fibrous bands and tongue flap reconstruction
   4. Selective tooth extraction.
   5. Obturator: Forced opening of jaws using screw obturator between upper and lower teeth.

Chronic Tonsillitis

An 8-year-old child presented with history of recurrent sore throat associated with fever for 2 years. Examination reveals enlarged faucial tonsils protruding towards midline (Figs 1A and B). Margins of anterior pillars is red. On pressing the anterior pillar whitish yellowish material comes out of the crypts. Jugulodigastric lymph nodes are hugely enlarged.

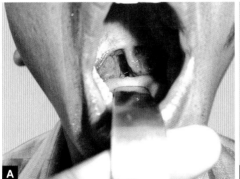 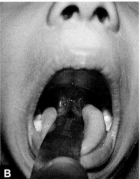

Figs 1A and B: (A) Enlarged tonsils; (B) Hugely enlarged (kissing tonsil)

Provisional Diagnosis: Chronic Tonsillitis

Q.1 What is chronic tonsillitis?
Ans. It is chronic infection of the faucial tonsils, which either results from recurrent acute tonsillitis or long-term infection of the tonsil.

Q.2 What are the points favorable of the diagnosis?
Ans. 1. History of recurrent attack of sore throat with fever.
   2. Hugely enlarged tonsils (Figs 1A and B).
   3. Anterior pillars are flushed, i.e. hyperemic margins.
   4. Irwin Moore's sign is positive: On pressing the anterior pillars pus or white yellowish purulent exudate with an offensive smell comes out of the crypts (water thin fluid may be lymph seen in normal subjects).
   5. Cervical (tonsillar glands), i.e. jugulodigastric lymph node are large and palpable (In 75% of normal children, cervical lymph nodes are palpable).

Q.3 Are tonsils always enlarged in chronic tonsillitis?

Ans. Not necessarily. Two varities are commonly seen:
1. Chronic parenchymatous: Tonsils are enlarged, usually seen in children and adolescents.
2. Chronic fibrotic: Common in adults, here the tonsils are fibrotic and adherent.

Q.4 What are other minor complaints that may be present in chronic tonsillitis?

Ans. 1. History of recurrent episodes of sore throat and fever.
2. Hawking and chowking may occur.
3. Unpleasant taste or smell from cheesy material.
4. Dysphagia or slow-eating habits due to hugely-enlarged tonsils.
5. Constant desire to clear up the throat.
6. Irritating cough.
7. Anorexia.
8. Weight loss.
9. Dyspnea.
10. Snoring:obstructive sleep apnea leading to corpulmonale in hugely-enlarged tonsils.
11. Development of change in temperaments, e.g. frequent irritation, bouts of cry for little reasons.
12. Lack of usual vigour.
13. Change in speech: Child may talk as his mouth is full (in case of enlarged tonsils.)

Q.5 What are the complications of tonsillitis?

Ans. Chronic tonsillitis if not treated may cause the following:
1. Recurrent acute tonsillitis.
2. Peritonsillitis and peritonsillar abscess.
3. Retropharyngeal and parapharyngeal space abscess.
4. Cervical lymphadenitis and cellulitis.
5. Laryngeal edema.
6. Otitis media.
7. Septicemia.
8. Sleep apnea.
9. Septic foci for—rheumatic fever, subacute bacterial endocarditis, nephritis, rheumatic chorea, arthritis.

Q.6 What is treatment of chronic tonsillitis?

Ans. Tonsillectomy—by various procedures, such as:
1. Dissection tonsillectomy (Waught)
2. Guillotine method.
3. Laser tonsillectomy—KTP-532 laser is used. It reduces intraoperative bleeding.
4. Cryosurgery.
5. Coblation tonsillectomy.
6. Radiofrequency tonsillectomy.

Q.7 What are the indications of tonsillectomy?

Ans. Indications of tonsillectomy are as follows:

1. Obstructive disease of tonsils:
   a. Obstructive to airway causing cor pulmonale
   b. Obstructive to food passage (mechanical) leading to weight loss
   c. Both or sleep apnoea syndrome.
2. Infections of tonsils:
   a. Peritonsillar abscess (after 4–6 weeks): Interval tonsillectomy
   b. Repeated attacks of acute tonsillitis (6 attacks a year for at least two years).
   c. Chronic tonsillitis.
3. Neoplasia tumor or tumorous conditions:
   a. Ulcer on tonsil suspician of malignancy (tonsillectomy biopsy)
   b. Unilateral enlarged tonsil with suspician of malignancy (sarcoma)
   c. Benign tumor specially sessile, e.g. fibroma, papilloma, lymphangioma, hemartoma (tonsil is removed with tumor mass).
4. Tonsil as a septic focus:
   a. Focus for persistant cervical lymphadenitis.
   b. Tubercular lymphadenitis.
   c. Recurrent pharyngitis or ear infection.
5. Septic focus for distant manifestation:
   a. Rheumatic fever or subcute bacterial endocarditis
   b. Acute glomerular nephritis.
   c. Arthritis, fibrositis, dermatitis.
6. As a route or approach to adjoining lesion:
   a. Glossopharyngeal neuralgia—for sectioning the nerve.
   b. Elongated styloid process surgery in Eagle's disease.
   c. For peritonsillar space or parapharyngeal space or for deep lobe of parotid gland.
7. As a persistant carriers:
   a. Streptococcus hemolyticus.
   b. Diphtheria.
   c. Other infection.
8. General diseases:
   a. General debility.
   b. Failure to gain weight.
   c. Malaise.
9. Before the other operation as a part:
   a. Undergoing palatopharyngoplasty.
   b. Before cleft palate surgery.
   c. Branchial fistula—to remove the complete tract.
10. Uncommon diseases of tonsils:
    a. Tonsillolith.
    b. Foreign body in tonsil.
    c. Tonsillar cyst.

11. Miscellaneous diseases:
   a. Trauma to tonsil.
   b. Intratonsillar hemorrhage.
   c. Gangrine.

Q.8 What are the contraindications of tonsillectomy?
Ans. Contraindications are: (Mnemonic ABCD....OP)
   A. Acute infection of the tonsil,pharynx and URI (3–4 weeks): Increased risk of hemorrhage and anesthesia.
   B. Bleeding disorder—hemophilia, purpura, leukemia.
   C. Cleft palate. chronic allergy.
   D. Diabetes.
   E. Epidemic of poliomyelitis.
   F. Febrile conditions and infections, fever, e.g. mumps, measles, chickenpox, typhoid, etc.
   G. Gastation or pregnancy.
   H. Hypertension.
   I. Internal carotid artery aneurysm.
   J. Jocker and singers specially classical singers.
   K. Kid less than 4 years.
   L. Low hemoglobin—less than 10 g%.
   M. Menstrual period.
   O. Oral contraceptives—cause more chances of deep vein thrombosis after tonsillectomy.
   P. Pulmonary tuberculosis—active lesion.

Q.9 Why tonsillectomy is contraindicated in child less than 4 years ?
Ans. 1. Average blood loss during routine tonsillectomy and adenoidectomy is between 100 and 130 mL (in adenoidectomy 60–77 of it get lost). Blood volume of a child is less than an adult. Blood volume of a child is calculated as 75 mL per kg body weight. During operation, blood loss is about 14%, so blood transfusion is usually required.
   2. Immunity development may be disturbed as functions of tonsils goes away.

Q.10 What are the procedures to assess the patient for pre-tonsillectomy?
Ans. 1. History of recurrent tonsillitis:
      a. Six attacks in a year for atleast 2 years;
      b. Sleep apnea.
   2. Clinical examination:
      a. Large tonsil;
      b. Large jugulodigastric lymph nodes.
   3. Bacteriological examination for culture and sensitivity.
   4. Serological tests—activated IgG and IgA are found in children with recurrent tonsillitis.
   5. Recurrent otitis media is an indicator.

Q.11 What are the investigations done before tonsillectomy ?

Ans. 1. General medical checkup—to exclude chest, kidney and liver diseases.

2. Hematological examination Hb, TLC, DLC, BT, CT, ESR, PT.

3. Urine analysis—for albumin, sugar and microscopic examination.

4. Blood for sugar, urea, creatinine.

5. X-ray chest PA view.

6. ECG.

Q.12 What are the postoperative care after tonsillectomy?

Ans. 1. Child should lie on the side with the head below the level of the shoulders.

2. Regular pulse-rate recording (every 15 minutes for first 2 hours, every 30 minutes for the next 2 hours, every 30 minutes for next 2 hours and hourly thereafter)

3. Close observation of breathing pattern.

4. Repeated examination of pharynx for hemorrhage.

5. Control of postoperative pain:Paracetamol.

Q.13 What are the indicators suggesting to post-tonsillectomy hemorrhage?

Ans. These are:

1. Audible noise on respiration is suggestive of blood in the pharynx in semiconscious child.

2. Excessive swallowing movements.

3. Vomiting of blood.

4. Rapid rising pulse.

5. A child looking increasingly grey in color or pale.

Q.14 What are the steps of dissection tonsillectomy?

Ans. 1. General anesthesia with orotracheal intubation and packing around the tube.

2. Rose position—supine position with extension of neck by keeping sand bag under the shoulders.

3. Exposure of the tonsils by opening the mouth with the help of Draffin's bipod rods and Boyle–Davis mouth gag.

4. Tonsil is held and pulled medially by Dennis Browne tonsil holding forceps or Andrew's tonsil valsellum.

5. Hockey-shaped incision is made by tonsillar knife or blade No. 15 at the upper pole mucosa with a cut in the semilunar fold.

6. Tonsil is dissected by making a cleavage between upper pole and tonsillar fossa.

7. Now the upper pole is held with Mukh's forceps or Dennis Browne forceps and rest of body of tonsil up to lower pole is dissected from its bed by cotton ball caught with Waugh dissection forceps or also with help of Mollison or tonsil dissector.

8. When the lower attachment (falsiform ligament) is reached Evans tonsil snare is used to crush and cut the pedicle.

9. Tonsillar fossa is then packed with rollar gauze or cotton balls and other side tonsil is removed.

10. Complete hemostasis—is achieved by catching the bleeding points with Burkitt's straight and then with curved forceps or with Wilson or Negus forceps. The ligature is tied (if required with the help of Negus knot tier) or small bleeding points may be cauterized with diathermy.

Q.15 What is postoperative treatment?
Ans. 1. Tonsillar position—left latreral position with knee and hip flexed.
2. Watch for bleeding.
3. Nothing by mouth for 6 hours.
4. Monitoring of PTR.
5. Analgesic.
6. Antibiotics.
7. Antiseptic gargles or weak hydrogen peroxide gargles.
8. Feeding as advised:
   – First 48 hours—ice cubes, cold things like ice cream and cold drinks.
   – After 48 hours—semisolid diet and soft diet.
   – After 72 hours—normal diet but without chillies and spice.
   – After 12-15 days—normal diet, chillies and spicy is allowed.

Q.16 What are postoperative complications after tonsillectomy?
Ans. 1. Hemorrhage (2.5%): Primary, reactionary and secondary.
2. Pulmonary complications.
3. Dental injury.
4. Posterior pillar and palatal injury.
5. Incomplete removal.
6. Acute otitis media.
7. Sepsis—retropharyngeal abscess/laryngeal edema.
8. Tight palate.
9. Speech changes.
10. Lingual tonsillitis, chronic grannular pharyngitis.

Q.17 Why cold drinks and ice cream are given for first 24 hours after tonsillectomy?
Ans. As the nerve endings are exposed causing cold anesthesia.

Q.18 Why lukewarm liquids are given after 24 hours following tonsillectomy?
Ans. As the inflammation starts; so the warm is always soothing for inflammation.

Q.19 How hydrogen peroxide is helpful followig tonsillectomy?
Ans. When hydrogen peroxide comes in contact with slough, there is release of nascent oxygen which helps in contraction blood vessels expelling small clots thereby causing closure of mouth of blood vessel, thus bleeding stops.

Q.20 What is reactionary hemorrhage and what are the causes in the tonsillectomy operation?

Ans. Reactionary hemorrhage can occur within 48 hours (approximately in about 1% of tonsillectomy; about 80% occurs in 24 hours).

The various causes are as follows:

1. Postoperative risk of rise in BP.
2. Slipping of ligature.
3. Clot in the fossa—which prevents retraction and contraction of blood vessels.
4. Failure to control proper primary hemorrhage.

Q.21 How will you manage the reactionary hemorrhage?

Ans. 1. Recording the vital parameters.
2. IV fluids and blood transfusion.
3. If the clot is small or dry—no surgical intervention is required.
4. If the clot is wet and excessive or active bleeding is present then:
   a. Shift the patient in OT.
   b. Controlling by gauze pressure.
   c. Ligation of bleeding points.
   d. Diathermy cauterization.
   e. Gauze pressure in fossa and suturing of pillars.

Q.22 What are the causes of secondary hemorrhages and how it is controlled in tonsillectomy operation?

Ans. Secondary hemorrhage is mainly due to infection. It occurs on 5th–7th day. Tonsillar fossa shows unhealthy slough. It occurs in about 1.2–1.5% of total operations. About 25% of these may require blood transfusion. Secondary hemorrhage is treated as follows:

1. Change of antibiotics: Massive dose of broad-spectrum antibiotics.
2. Local pressure.
3. Blood transfusion.
4. Antiseptic gargle.
5. Suturing of anterior and posterior pillars.
6. Carotid (external) artery ligation (if above measures fail).

Q. 23 If hemorrhage is suspected in post-tonsillectomy period, what steps should be taken?

Ans. 1. IV patency maintenance.
2. Blood for crossmatching.
3. Baseline hemoglobin estimation.
4. BP monitoring with PTR.
5. Preparation for anesthesia—experienced anesthetist is required as re-anesthesia is hazardous.

Enlarged Adenoids

CASE: A child of 6 years of age presents with typical adenoid facies. Postnasal mirror examination reveals an enlarged adenoid mass in the nasopharynx.

Provisional Diagnosis: Enlarged Adenoids

Q.1 What is adenoids?

Ans. Adenoids are one of the members of Waldeyer's ring and are also called pharyngeal tonsil of Luschka. It is a submucosal collection of lymphoid tissue at the roof and posterior wall of the nasopharynx. It is a single midline structure having vertical ridges (usually 6–8 in number). It has neither crypts nor capsule. It gets atrophied at the age of puberty. In the center of lymphoid mass, there is depression called "pharyngeal bursa". Thornwald's cyst develops from this bursa.

Q.2 When do the adenoids become pathological?

Ans. When the adenoids produce effect either due to infection (adenoiditis) or due to hypertrophy or enlargement. Size of adenoids relative to the nasopharynx, is more important rather than adenoid size, to produce symptoms.

Q.3 What are the effects of enlarged adenoids?

Ans. Enlarged adenoids can give rise to symptoms in relation to various systems like:
1. Nasal symptoms.
2. Ear symptoms.
3. Adenoid facies.
4. Oral symptoms.
5. General manifestations.

Q.4 What are various nasal symptoms in relation to enlarged adenoids?

Ans. Most of the nasal symptoms are due to nasal obstruction, nasal block, nasal discharge, mouth breathing, evidence of sinusitis change in voice (Rhinolalia clausa), nasal intonation or toneless voice, noisy respiration, wet bubbly nose, postnasal discharge, headache and recurrent epistaxis.

Q.5 What are ear-related symptoms in enlarged adenoids?

Ans. Ear symptoms are due to Eustachian tube obstruction, recurrent acute otitis media and otitis media with effusion (glue ear), earache off and on, conductive deafness and chronic suppurative otitis media.

Q.6 What are various oral symptoms in adenoids?

Ans. Oral symptoms are mouth breathing, slow eating (long time taken in meals) swollowing unchewed or partially chewed food, dribbling of saliva, retracted upper lip, sore at the angle of mouth, narrowing of the maxillary arch, crowding of teeth and protruding out of upper teeth, high-arched palate, snoring at night and dryness of tongue.

Q.7 What are various facial features manifested in enlarged adenoids?

Ans. Facial feature that constitutes adenoid fancies are as follows:
1. Dull expressionless face.
2. Idiotic look.
3. Pinched nose.
4. Open mouth (an open-lip posture).
5. Less prominent nasolabial sulcus, nonfunctioning ala nasi.
6. Constant running of the nose with stasis over upper lip.
7. Dribbling of saliva through angle of mouth.
8. Short upper lip.
9. Protruded teeth.
10. Narrow maxillary arch.
11. Higharched palate.
12. Hypoplastic maxilla.
13. Either upper jaw protruded or lower jaw recedes.
14. Occlusion abnormalities.

Q.8 What are the main features of adenoid facies?

Ans. 1. An open-lip posture with prominent upper teeth and short upper lip.
2. A thin nose with hypoplastic maxilla, narrow upper alveolus and high-arched palate.

Q.9 What are other conditions in which these features can be observed?

Ans. 1. Child with persistent thumb sucking.
2. Child with use of dummy.
3. Habitual mouth breather.
4. Inherited hypoplastic maxilla.

Q.10 What is sleep apnea?

Ans. It is characterized by apneic episodes during sleep associated by hypersomnolence during day when person has at least 30 episodes of apnoea lasting 10 seconds or more during 6 hours of sleep which are associated with hypoxemia or bradycardia.

Sleep apnea may be:
1. Obstruction sleep apnea: When the symptoms of sleep apnea is produced by obstruction to upper airway.
2. Central apnea: If the cause of sleep apnea is in the brain.

These may induce the following:
1. Ventricular failure
2. Pulmonary edema and pulmonary infection
3. Cor pulmonale
4. Day-time sleepiness

Q.11 What are various investigations for sleep apnea?
Ans. 1. Clinically: Snoring, noisy breathing even when child is awake, day time sleepiness
2. Investigations are as follows:
   a. Radiological: Soft tissue nasopharynx (lateral view)
   b. Polysomnography: It monitors brain activity, eye movements, heart rate, and chest movements
   c. Earlobe oxymetry for oxygen saturation recording.

Q.12 What are general manifestations for enlarged adenoids?
Ans. Various general manifestations are as follows:
1. Pharynx—recurrent pharyngitis, tonsillitis.
2. Larynx—recurrent laryngitis, laryngis stridulous, snoring, nocturnal cough.
3. Inability to concentrate (Grey's approsexia), mentally weak, back bencher in school.
4. Respiratory system—consistently vulnerable for upper respiratory infection (URI) and lower respiratory tract infection (LRI).
5. Effect on chest development; pigeons chest, Harrison's sulcus (Fig. 1)
6. Abdomen—pot bellied.
7. Nutrition—anemia, malnutrition, stunted growth.
8. Neck—enlarged neck lymph nodes (chain at the posterior border of sternomastoid muscle).
9. Reflexes—nocturnal enuresis, insomnia.
10. Gastroenteritis, malabsorption, recurrent diarrhea due to unchewed food and swallowing of ingested discharge.

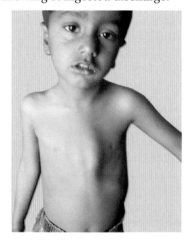

Fig. 1: Chest effect of adenoid (pegion's chest)

Q.13 What are the indications of adenoidectomy?

Ans. Following are the indications of adenoidectomy:

1. Nasal obstruction—a narrow airway obstruction assessed by clinical examination and radiography.
2. Otitis media with effusion.
3. Recurrent acute otitis media.
4. Sleep apnea.

Q.14 What are the contraindications of adenoidectomy?

Ans. 1. Acute infection—recurrent URI.
2. Bleeding disorders.
3. Cleft palate—cleft palate, congenital short palate or submucous cleft palate.
4. General diseases.

Q.15 What are the various methods used for examining the adenoids?

Ans. Adenoids can be examined by the following methods:

1. Postnasal mirror examination—in cooperative elder child.
2. Digital examination under general anesthesia (GA).
3. Nasal endoscopy (Fig. 2).
4. X-ray lateral view of the nasopharynx (Figs 3A and B).
5. Flexible nasopharyngoscopy.
6. Computed tomography (CT) and magnetic resonance imaging (MRI).

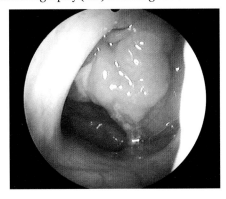

Fig. 2: Endoscopic view of enlarged adenoid

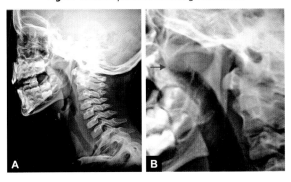

Figs 3A and B: X-ray nasopharynx (lateral view): Enlarged adenoid

Q.16 What are the steps of adenoidectomy?

Ans. 1. Patient should be under deep GA with absent pharyngeal reflex otherwise contraction of superior constrictor muscle would not allow adenoid removal in precision.
   2. Natural position of the neck—not hyperextension otherwise tearing of pharyngeal mucosa.
   3. Digital examination of nasopharynx with index finger.
   4. Mouth is kept opened with Boyle's Davi's mouth gag.
   5. Insertion of a St. Clair Thombson's curette (guarded, i.e. with teeth) in to the nasopharynx gently positioned against the posterior end of nasal septum.
   6. This appropriate size is swept downwards, curetting the adenoid mass.
   7. As the mass of adenoid is curetted the blade of the curette is brought forward to avoid running it down the posterior wall and stripping mucosa.
   8. The remnant are removed by simple curette repeatedly or avulsed by Luc's forceps (direction of avulsion is cranial otherwise pharyngeal mucosa will be stripped).
   9. Digital palpation of nasopharyngeal is done again for any tag of residual mass which is curetted out if any.
   10. Pack is than placed into nasopharynx to help hemostasis. A second pack is kept for 5 minutes.
   11. Airway patency: Clear the airway aspiration of blood and secretions by catheter suction.

Q.17 What are the complications of adenoid surgery?

Ans. Complications are as follows:
   1. Excessive hemorrhage:
      a. Primary—causes are coagulopathy, trauma, localized hypofibrinogenemia, aberrant vessels, and injury to pharyngeal plexus. Treatment is diathermy cautry, removal of remnant and postnasal packing.
      b. Reactionary—causes are hypertension, remnant. Treatment is removal of remnant, diathermic cautery, postnasal packing and blood transfusion.
      c. Secondary—cause is infection
      Treatment is change of antibiotics to broad spectrum and postnasal packing.
   2. Surgical trauma—to soft palate, eustachian tube cushion (stenosis later on), dislocation of cervical spines.
   3. Effect on speech—hypernasal speech.
   4. Scarring of fibrous bands or adhesion in nasopharynx.
   5. Pulmonary complications (due to anesthesia): Aspiration, collapse, abscesses.
   6. Secretory otitis media (rare).
   7. Traumatic granuloma.

Q.18 Why digital palpation of the nasopharynx is done before adenoidectomy?

Ans. Digital palpation with index finger is done to:
1. Confirm the size of adenoid mass (palpation is felt like "worms in bag").
2. To dissect and bring the lateral extension of adenoid to midline.
3. To ascertain the position of Eustachian tube.
4. To feel for any abnormal pulsation, i.e. any abnormal vessel.

Q.19 What are the causes of persistence of symptoms following adenoid surgery?

Ans. 1. The adenoid was not responsible for symptoms.
2. Postoperative scarring in nasopharynx or at the opening of Eustachian tube.
3. Remnant of lymphoid tissue in the nasopharynx following incomplete removal.
4. Hypertrophy of same remnant of the lymphoid tissue.

Vocal Cord Nodules (Singer's Nodule)

CASE: Patient presented with hoarseness of voice which worsens by evening due to fatigue for a month duration. Indirect laryngoscopy shows pinkish white nodules at the junction of anterior one-third and posterior two-third (Fig. 1).

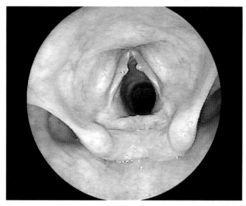

Fig. 1: Vocal cord nodules

Provisional Diagnosis: Vocal Cord Nodules

Q.1 What is vocal nodule?
Ans. It is also called singers or screamer nodes. It consists of localized epithelial hyperplastic lesion of the free edge of vocal cords usually at the junction of anterior one-third due to misuse or abuse of the voice.

Q.2 What are the predisposing factors?
Ans. 1. More common in females of age between 20 and 30 years.
2. It can also occur in children.
3. Misuse or abuse of voice.
4. It is common in teachers, actors, vendors, or pop singers.

Q.3 What is the pathogenesis of vocal cord nodules?
Ans. 1. The anterior part is the site for maximum vibration so at the junction of anterior one-third and posterior two-thirds, more friction occurs during faulty use of voice which results in localized exudation and fibrosis and thus, nodule formation.

2. Vocal nodules results due to hyperkertosis at vocal cords in response to excessive strain by producing a 'submucosal hemorrhage' underlying fibrosis and some cell infiltration.

Q.4 What is the differential diagnosis?

Ans. All cases of hoarseness of voice in particular:

1. Chronic laryngitis
2. Papilloma
3. Polyps
4. Keratosis
5. Tuberculosis
6. Syphilis.

Q.5 What is the treatment?

Ans. 1. Voice rest.
2. Avoid misuse and abuse of voice (singing should be corrected).
3. Smoking should be avoided.
4. Surgery—microlaryngoscopic excision.
5. Speech therapy.
6. Scalping by laser.

Q.6 What are the various stages and their treatment?

Ans. 1. Early or soft nodules resolve with speech therapy and good vocal habits.
2. Long established (hard) nodule require microsurgical excision.

Q.7 Why is it called singer's nodule?

Ans. It is a disease of professional voice user.

1. Chiefly singing in high-range.
2. High-tone in faulty manner.
3. Singing beyond their natural range.
4. Coup de glotte (glottic shock technique) cords come together in an abnormally violent manner.
5. Vocal abuse—too frequently repeated.
6. When the cords does not vibrate as a whole but in segment depending on the pitchs of the cord during singing and speaking, i.e. anterior portion is active while posterior is inert.

CASE

42

Vocal Cord Polyp

CASE: Patients presents with hoarseness of voice for some duration. Indirect laryngoscopy shows a single, smooth, pink and pedunculated mass arising from one cord.

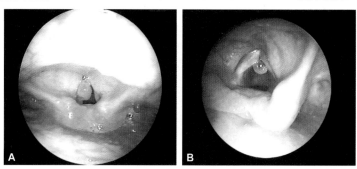

Figs 1 and B: (A) Vocal cord polyp; (B) Vocal polyp at anterior commissure

Provisional Diagnosis: Vocal Cord Polyp

Q.1 What are predisposing factors?
Ans. It may be due to allergy, trauma, hematoma, chronic infection, smoking.

Q.2 What is the treatment?
Ans. Microlaryngoscopic excision.

Q.3 How vocal cord polyp is formed ?
Ans. Localized vascular engorgement and microhemorrhages followed by edema. Polyp is fluid-filled swelling or bumb or blister-like lesion (Reinke's edema).

Q.4 What are the features of vocal cord polyp?
Ans. It can be translucent (Fig. 1A), reddish or pedunculated lesion usually arising from vocal cord in anterior half common near anterior commissure (Fig. 1B). It may hung down into subglottic region and visible on coughing or phonation.

Q.5 What is the difference between vocal cord polyp and cyst?
Ans. The cysts are intracordal whereas polyps are pedunculated and may hung down on their stalk to sit below the cords.

Contact Ulcer Larynx

CASE: Patient presents with hoarseness of voice and pain in throat of 10-month duration. Indirect laryngoscopy shows heaped edge of vocal process of one side which may appear fitting in a grater of the opposite cord giving an appearness of ulcer.

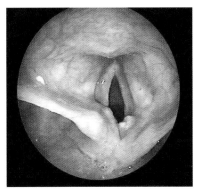

Fig. 1: A raised nodular mass at the vocal process region

Provisional Diagnosis: Contact Ulcer Larynx

Q.1 What is contact ulcer?

Ans. It was described by C Jackson. So also called contact ulcer of Jackson. Actually these are not ulcers. It is contact pachydermia resulting from misuse of voice. The lesions appear on the vocal process. The localized thickened hyperplastic epithelium gets headed up around a crater. There may be granuloma formation (Fig. 1).

Q.2 What is the treatment?

Ans. 1. Voice rest.
  2. Proper speech therapy.
  3. Microlaryngoscopy excision.
  4. Treatment of acid reflex.

Q.3 What is the pathogenesis?

Ans. A localized thickened hyperplastic epithelium occurring on the vocal process without involving the membranous portion of vocal cords. Thicking occurs in a form of oval mound on the inner surface of vocal cords but extending also on its upper surface (due to the hammering of one vocal process to another).

Q.4 Why does patient develop change in voice?

Ans. 1. On phonation, the localized heaped up area (mounds) comes into contact and prevents complete adduction of the cords.

2. Due to repeated striking of one mound with the other mound of the vocal process, a grater-like depression is formed on one mound.

3. On phonation characteristic "cup and ball" filling of the mounds is seen. Thus vocal fatigue and hoarseness of voice are chief symptoms.

44 Unilateral Vocal Cord Paralysis

CASE: A patient presents with hoarseness of voice of sudden onset. Indirect laryngoscopy reveals paramedian position of left vocal cord which does not move laterally even on deep inspiration (Fig. 1B).

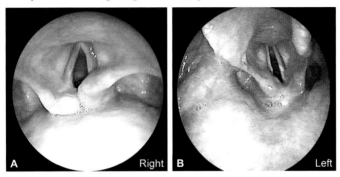

Figs 1A and B: (A) Right vocal cord paralysis; (B) Left vocal cord paralysis

Provisional Diagnosis: Unilateral Vocal Cord Paralysis

Q.1 What is characteristic of voice in vocal cord palsy?

Ans. Patient has a week breathy voice rather than the harsh hoarseness of voice which is characteristic of laryngeal cancer. Patient has a poor, ineffective cough and with associated tendency of aspiration.

Q.2 What are causes of impaired movement of the vocal cord?

Ans. Vocal cord mobility can be impaired by the defect in the muscle itself (fibrosis, infiltration by growth, weight of growth), myoneural junction affection, cricoarytenoid joint pathology (rheumatoid arthritis or growth infiltrating the joint, or inflammatory diseases, fibrosis), or due to recurrent laryngeal nerve paralysis (Figs 1A and B).

Q.3 What are different positions of vocal cords?

Ans. 1. Position remain in median position in normal phonation and in recurrent laryngeal nerve palsy.
2. Paramedian position (1.5 mm away): Normally in strong whisper and in reccurent laryngeal nerve palsy (Figs 1A and B).

3. Intermediate (Cadaveric) position (3.5 mm away for midline). This is neutral position of cricoarytenoid joint. Abduction and adduction take place from this position. This cadaveric position with impaired mobility is seen in paralysis of both recurrent laryngeal nerve (also where recurrent and superior laryngeal nerve get paralyzed).
4. Gentle abduction (7 mm away) is on quite respiration and also in adduction paralysis.
5. Full abduction (95 mm away) is during deep inspiration.

Q.4 Why does the vocal cord assume the median or paramedian position in case of recurrent laryngeal palsy?

Ans. Recurrent laryngeal nerve supplies all the intrinsic muscles of the larynx (abductors and adductors) except the cricothyroid muscle (supplied by superior laryngeal nerve). Median or paramedian position is due to:
1. Semon's law states that in all progressive organic lesions abductor fibers of the nerve (which is phylogenetically newer) are more susceptible and so first paralyzed than the fibers of adductors.
2. Wagner and Grossmen hypothesis: It is due to intact function of cricothyroid muscle which is innervated by the superior laryngeal nerve.

Q.5 What are the causes of recurrent laryngeal nerve palsy?

Ans. Causes of right and left recurrent laryngeal nerve palsy are different as the right recurrent laryngeal nerve passes into the neck and take a turn around the subclavian artery while the left recurrent laryngeal nerve passes into the mediastinum and then take a turn around the arch of aorta.
1. Causes of right recurrent laryngeal nerve paralysis in the neck:
   - Trauma.
   - Thyroid disease
   - Thyroid surgery.
   - Carcinoma cervical esophagus.
   - Cervical lymphadenopathy.
   - Aneurysm of subclavian artery.
   - Carcinoma of apex of right lung.
   - Tuberculosis of cervical pleura.
   - Iodiopathic.
2. Causes of paralysis of left recurrent laryngeal nerve:
   - Causes in the neck:
     - Accidental trauma.
     - Thyroid disease.
     - Carcinoma of cervical esophagus.
     - Cervical lymphadenopathy.
     - Thyroid surgery.
   - Causes in the mediastinum: Cancer lung, carcinoma of thoracic esophagus, aortic aneurysm, mediastinal lymphadenopathy, intrathoracic surgery, enlarged left auricle, i.e mitral stenosis (Ortner's syndrome).

- Causes of both recurrent laryngeal nerve paralysis:
  - Thyroid surgery.
  - Carcinoma thyroid.
  - Carcinoma of cervical esophagus.
  - Cervical lymphadenopathy.
- Miscellaneous causes: Rheumatoid arthritis, collagen vascular disorder, hemolytic anemia, syphilis, diphtheria.

Q.6 What is treatment of recurrent laryngeal nerve (RLN) palsy?

Ans. Usually no treatment is required. The voice may gradually improve due to compensation by the healthy cord which crosses the midline to approximate with paralyzed cord.

In some cases which do not recover even after several years, surgery is required:

1. Phonosurgery: Medialization of the vocal cord
2. Glottic rehabilitation with Teflon injection.
3. Arytenoids rotation.
4. RLN reinnervation.

Q.7 What are the features of paralysis of superior laryngeal nerve?

Ans. 1. Voice is weak and pitch cannot be raised.
   2. Unilateral anesthesia of larynx (supraglottic) usually does not causes aspiration.
   3. Larynged finding: Due to cricothyroid muscles.
      a. Askew position of glottic are oblique-glottic. Anterior commissure rotates to the healthy side and the posterior commissure to the side of paralysis.
      b. Shortening of cord with loss of tension.
      c. Wavy appearance of cord with low level (levels differences of the cord)
      d. Flapping: Vocal sags down during inspiration and goes up during inspiration.
   4. Chronic repeated aspiration may require surgical procedure, e.g epiglottopexy or teflon injection for medialization.

Q.8 What are the common causes of bilateral adductor palsy?

Ans. Causes are:

1. Functional
2. Early tubercular.

Flag sign is seen in such cases, voice is weak and husky.

Q.9 What are the causes of neurological disorders of larynx?

Ans. 1. Supra nuclear—rare.
   2. Nuclear—medullary tumor, syringobulbia, motor neuron disease.

3. High val lesions (combined paralysis), posterior fossa tumor, benign meningitis, skull base fracture, nasopharyngeal cancer. Glomus tumor, parapharyngeal masses and metastatic disease.
4. Superior laryngeal nerve palsy: Thyroid surgery, penetrating neck trauma, diphtheria, metastatic cervical adenopathy.
5. Recurrent laryngeal nerve palsy.

Q.10 What investigations to be done in vocal cord palsy?
Ans. Rules of third:
1. Idiopathic (One-third)
2. Surgery (One-third)
3. Neoplasia (One-third).
Thus investigations are (history of operation is negative then):
1. X-ray chest PA view
2. CT scan skull to hilum
3. USG
4. Esophagoscopy.
If the above are negative then postviral neuropathy is likely to be the cause.

Q.11 What are differentiating points between paralysis and fixed vocal cord?
Ans.

Paralysis	Fixed vocal cord
Bowing of the cord	Cord is straight and looks shortened
Medial deviation of arytenoids cartilage on affected side	Position of arytenoids according to condition causing fixation
Flicker of vocal cord on phonation	No flicker
On probe test, the paralytic cord shows vibration	No vibration

Q.12 What are causes of vocal cord immobility (fixation of cord)?
Ans. The causes are:
1. Rheumatoid arthritis.
2. Laryngeal trauma.
3. Prolonged intubation.
4. Cancer involving the cricoarytenoid joint.

Juvenile Multiple Papilloma Larynx

CASE: A 3-year-old child was brought by the parents with history of hoarseness of voice from 6 months and respiratory distress for the last one week.

Provisional Diagnosis: Juvenile Multiple Papilloma of the Larynx

Q.1 What is juvenile multiple papilloma of larynx?
Ans. These are recurrent respiratory papilloma caused by human papilloma virus 6 and 11.

Q.2 What is human papillomavirus ?
Ans. It is a small DNA virus 50 nm in diameter. There are over 70 types of human papillomavirus. It is the same virus that causes warts on the penis, vulva, cervix and perianal areas.

After infection, the virus remains in basal layer of the mucous membrane as episomal maintenance under dormant so can recur after several years of remission.

Q.3 What is epidemiology of JM papilloma?
Ans. 1. Age before 14: Female preponderance.
2. Age after 14: Male preponderance.
3. Age onset from 6 month to 1 year.
4. Majority of children present before the age 4 years.
5. Age less than 5 years: 60% probability of mother having genital wart at the time of delivery.
6. Transmitted at the time of delivery.
7. Route of transmission is through inhalation.
8. There may be some defect in hot immune system.

Q.4 What are presenting symptoms?
Ans. 1. Hoarseness of voice or an abnormal cry (initial symptom).
2. Increasing stridor (late manifestation).
3. Acute respiratory obstruction (rare).

Q.5 What are the sites for multiple papilloma larynx?

Ans. 1. Early lesions commonly at anterior aspect of the glottic and anterior commissure (point of airway narrowing)—postpart is not affected because of protective mechanism of thick mucous blanket and more rapid rate of its movement. False cords and epiglottic also affected.

   2. Late lesions: Later on whole larynx is involved as the disease advances and protective normal flow of mucous blanket is disrupted.

   3. Advanced lesion: Involvement of trachea after tracheostomy due to disruption of protective mucous blanket flow and airflow.

   4. Bronchial involvement: 2% of all patients eventually has bronchial lesion.

Q.6 What are the characteristics of the disease?

Ans. 1. Clusters of papilloma: Sessile, spread over a wide area of mucosa, or frible, bleed easily, may be pedunculated and localized.

   2. Unpredictable recurrence (due to presence of viral episome in apparently normal cells):

      a. Early recurrence: Within 2 weeks removal of papilloma has an enhancing effect on growth rate

      b. Recurrence may be larger than the original lesion

      c. There may be no recurrence for 5 or 20 years.

   3. Diffuse disease: Having papilloma at nostril (mucocutaneous junction), on gingiva and lips, both surface of soft palate and tonsillar pillars, in larynx, in tracheobronchial tree, and occasionally in the pulmonary parenchyma and at esophageal inlet.

   4. Multiple papilloma have a predilection for points of airway constriction where there is

      a. Increased airflow

      b. Drying

      c. Crusting and irritation.

Q.7 What are the effects of tracheotomy in multiple papilloma?

Ans. 1. Papilloma occurs around tracheotomy site.

   2. Papilloma occurs at the tip of tracheostomy tube.

   3. Explosive increase in tracheal papilloma.
      So tracheotomy should be avoided if it is possible to establish a normal airway by endoscopic removal of papilloma.

Q.8 What are the factors causing remission in multiple papilloma disease?

Ans. Remission can occur at any age usually at puberty and at any time irrespective of complete or incomplete removal or method of removal. The factors are as follows:

   1. Chance of remission is more, if disease present between age of 6–10 years.

   2. Patient with age of 16 years.

   3. Chances of remission, if treated by laser is 46%.

   4. Patient at or after 16 years—remission rate is 26%.

   5. Remission rate in larynx is 48, tracheobronchial tree 27% and in the lung 0%.
   6. Duration of remission—varies from 2 years to life long.

Q.9 How does multiple papilloma of the larynx spread lower down?
Ans. Spread to tracheobronchial tree is 11% and to lung parenchyma 3%.

Q.10 What is the finding in X-ray in case of spread of papilloma in the lungs?
Ans. Pulmonary spread is multicentric, progressive and eventually fatal, reveals cystic spaces which is filled with air or fluid.

Q.11 What are the chances of malignant degeneration in multiple papilloma of the larynx?
Ans. 1. Risk is extremely low.
   2. Risk is more if radiotherapy is given.
   3. Risk is more if patient is smoking.
   4. Malignant change may occur in adult, specially with subtypes 7 and 11.

Q.12 What is the treatment?
Ans. 1. Surgical extirpation (surgical debulking).
   2. Microelectrocautery.
   3. CO_2 laser vaporization—disadvantage:
      a. Scarring at anterior commissure and posterior commissure
      b. Chance of inhalation of smoke generated by laser.
   4. Cryosurgery.
   5. Extirpation using microdebrider.
   6. Medical treatment:
      a. Inosine pranobex, adenine ara benoside, lysozyme chlorhydrate.
      b. Antiviral agents: Acyclovir, ribavirin.
      c. Interferon is effective but rebound growth may be quick and several when it is stopped.

Q.13 What precautions should be taken during surgery?
Ans. To reduce scarring, care should be taken to try:
   1. To avoid damage to underlying and adjacent membrane.
   2. Avoid of exposure of vocalis muscle.

Q.14 Why the disease is difficult to treat or cure?
Ans. 1. Multifocal nature.
   2. Dormant virus episomes present in basal layer.
   3. High recurrence rate.
   4. Reduced immune competency.

Cancer Larynx

CASE: A 65-year-old man presented with history of progressive hoarsness of voice. He was habitual of smoking (30 years) and addicted to alcohol. Indirect laryngoscopy reveals a ulcerative growth involving the anterior-half of right vocal cord, anterior commissure and anterior one-third of the left vocal cord.

Provisional Diagnosis: Cancer Glottic Region

Q.1 What is the incidence of cancer larynx?
Ans. 1. It constitutes about 20% of all parts of malignancy.
　　2. Common in India than western countries.
　　3. Males affected more than female (10%).
　　4. Common in age group 40–70 years.

Q.2 What are its predisposing factors?
Ans. 1. Tobacco 2–3 times.
　　2. Alcohol 2–3 times.
　　3. Combination of tobacco and alcohol—increase the risk 18-folds.
　　4. Previous radiation.
　　5. Genetic factors.
　　6. Occupation exposure to asbestos, mustard gas, petroleum products.
　　7. Atmospheric pollutants.

Q.3 Why is carcinoma of the larynx classified on anatomical basis?
Ans. The larynx is divided into supraglottic, glottic and subglottic region. This division is based on drainage of lymphatic. The area above the vocal cord drains upward via superior lymphatic to upper deep cervical lymph nodes. The subglottic lymphatic drain to the prelaryngeal and tracheal lymph nodes.
　　These sites are subdivided (AJCC classification 1997) into the following:
　　1. Supraglottic:
　　　　– Suprahyoid epiglottis (both lingual and laryngeal surface)
　　　　– Infrahyoid epiglottis
　　　　– Aryepiglottic folds (laryngeal aspect only)

- Arytenoids
- Ventricular bands (or false cord)
- Ventricles and saccule
2. Glottis:
- True vocal cords including anterior and posterior commisure
3. Subglottic: Up to lower border of cricoid cartilage.

Q.4 What is TNM classification of larynx?
Ans. Cancer at each site is further classified by TNM system.

Q.5 Why did the fixity of lymph node dropped from TNM classification?
Ans. The term fixity is dropped as it involves as subjective element of variation, as it is seen generally more than 6 cm.

TNM Classification of Cancer Larynx (American Joint Committee on Cancer, 1997)

Supraglottis
T1: Tumor limited to one subsite of supraglottis with normal vocal cord mobility.
T2: Tumor invades mucosa of more than one adjacent subsite of supraglottis or region outside the supraglottis (e.g. mucosa of base of tongue, vallecula, medial wall of pyriform sinus) without fixation of the larynx.
T3: Tumor limited to larynx with vocal cord fixation and/or invades any of the following—postcricoid area, pre-epiglottic tissues.
T4: Tumor extends through the thyroid cartilage, and/or extends into soft tissue of the neck, thyroid and/or esophagus.

Glottis
T1: Tumor limited to vocal cord (may involve anterior or posterior commisures) with normal mobility.
T1a: Tumor limited to one vocal cord.
T1b: Tumor involves both vocal cords.
T2: Tumor extends to supraglottis and/or with impaired vocal cord mobility.
T3: Tumor limited to the larynx with vocal cord fixation.
T4: Tumor invades through thyroid cartilage and/or other tissues beyond the larynx, e.g. trachea, soft tissue of neck, including thyroid, pharynx.

Subglottis
T1: Tumor limited to the subglottis.
T2: Tumor extends to the vocal cord (s) with normal or impaired mobility.
T3: Tumor limited to the larynx with vocal cord fixation.
T4: Tumor invades through cricoid or thyroid cartilage and/or extends to other tissues beyond the larynx (e.g., trachea, soft tissues of neck, including thyroid, esophagus)

Regional lymph nodes (N)

Nx: Regional lymph nodes cannot be assessed.

N0: No regional lymph node metastasis.

N1: Metastasis in a single ipsilateral lymph node, 3 cm or less in greatest dimension.

N2: Metastasis in a single ipsilateral lymph node, more than 3 cm but not more than 6 cm in greatest dimension, or multiple ipsilateral lymph node, none more than 6 cm in greatest dimension, or bilateral or cotralateral lymph nodes, none more than 6 cm in greatest dimension.

N2a: Metastasis in a sigle ipsilateral lymph node more than 3 cm but not more than 6 cm in greatest dimension.

N2b: Metastasis in multiple ipsilateral lymph nodes, none more than 6 cm in greatest dimension.

N2c: Metastasis in bilateral or contralateral lymph nodes, none more than 6 cm in greatest dimension.

N3: Metastasis in a lymph node more than 6 cm in greatest dimension.

Distant metastasis (M)

Mx: Distant metastasis cannot be assessed.

M0: No distant metastasis.

M1: Distant metastasis.

Q.6 What is stage grouping for cancer larynx?

Ans. Stage grouping for cancer larynx is as follows:

0	Tis	N0	M0
I	T1	N0	M0
II	T2	N0	M0
III	T3	N0	M0
	T1	N1	M0
	T2	N1	M0
	T3	N1	M0
IVA	T4	N0	M0
	T4	N1	M0
	AnyT	N2	M0
IVB	AnyT	N3	M0
IVC	AnyT	AnyN	M1

Q.7 What is histological grading for cancer larynx?

Ans. Grade 1: Well-differentiated

Grade 2: Moderately differentiated

Grade 3: Poorly differentiated.

Q.8 What are the clinical features of supraglottic carcinoma?

Ans. 1. It is relatively less frequent (35%) and mainly involves the epiglottis, false cord followed by aryepiglottic fold.

2. Supraglottic growth are often silent.

3. Supraglottic cancer is usually anaplastic.

4. Earlist symptoms are dysphagia, throat pain, otalgia, mass of lymph nodes in the neck, foreign body sensation in throat or lump in throat.
5. Late symptoms are usually change in voice (Hot potato speech), hoarseness of voice (vocal cord is involved), cough, hemoptysis, halitosis, stridor and inspiratory dyspnea and weight loss.
6. Indirect laryngoscopy reveals a cauliflower like growth or an ulcer.
7. Pooling of secretion due to irritation and dysphagia.
8. Metastatic lymph node upper or middle group of deep jugular chain, initially firm then hard. Bilateral involvement, if growth crosses the midline.

Q.9 How does supraglottic cancer spread?

Ans. 1. It may spread locally and invades nearly areas, e.g. vallcula, posterior third tongue and pyriform fossa.
   – Extension to pre-epiglottic space from group of infrahyoid epiglottic, anterior ventricular band.
   – Penetrate the thyroid gland from pre-epiglottic space.
2. By lymphatic: Regional lymph node upper and middle deep cervical.
3. Hematogenoma: Rare to lungs, liver and bone.

Q.10 What are the features of glottic carcinoma?

Ans. 1. Most common site (60%) laryngeal cancer
2. Usually arises from the free margin of the upper surface of anterior third of vocal cord
3. Majority are squamous cell carcinoma, of cell differentiated
4. Hoarseness of voice is one of earliest symptoms.

Q.11 What are the various symptoms of glottic carcinoma?

Ans. 1. Early symptoms are: Hoarseness of voice, dry cough and raw sensation in throat.
2. Late symptoms are: Blood stained sputum, stridor, dyspnea, painful widening of larynx and palpable lymph nodes.

Q.12 How does a glottic carcinoma spread?

Ans. Localy, it spreads directly to the neighboring structures:
1. Forward to the anterior commissure and to the anterior portion of the opposite site.
2. Backward to arytenoids cartilage and interarytenoid region.
3. Upward, towards the ventricle.
4. Downward to the subglottic region.
5. Laterally towards the cartilage, leading to vocal cord fixation. It may lead to perichondritis with painful widening of the larynx.

Q.13 How does glottic cancer spread by lymphatic?

Ans. There are a few lymphatic in vocal cords, so nodal metastasis is rare. When the carcinoma spreads beyond the regional of membranous cord-metastasis occurs in prelaryngeal (Delphian's lymph node) and paratracheal lymph nodes, subsequently middle jugular nodes are involved.

Q.14 What are the clinical features of subglottic cancer?

Ans. 1. Subglottic carcinoma is rare (1–2%).
2. It involves the area from the inferior margin of the true vocal cord to the inferior run of cricoid.
3. Locally, it spreads downward to the trachea, upward to the vocal cord and circumferentially inside the larynx.
4. Metastasis occurs in pretracheal, paratracheal and mediastinal lymph nodes.
5. Stridor or respiratory distress is earliest symptom.
6. Hoarseness of voice is late feature.

Q.15 How does subglottic cancer produce hoarseness of voice?

Ans. 1. Spread of disease to under surface of vocal cords.
2. Infiltration to thyroarytenoid muscle.
3. Involvement of recurrent laryngeal nerve at cricoarytenoid joint.

Q.16 How will you make diagnosis cancer larynx?

Ans. 1. History: Symtomatology depends on site of origin whether it is glottic, supraglottic or subglottic. Dictum is any aged person having persistent or gradieralty increasing hoarseness of voice for 3 weeks must have laryngeal examination to exclude cancer.
2. Indirect larygoscopy due to node:
   a. Appearance of growth: Vary with site of origin:
      i. Suprahyoid epiglottis are usually exophytic (Figs 1B, C, E and F) while these of infrahyoid are ulcerative.
      ii. Lesion of vocal cord: usually raised nodule, ulcer or thickened area (Figs 1A and D).
      iii. Lesion of at anterior commissure as granulation tissue.
      iv. Subglottic lesion as a raised submucosal nodule, mostly on anterior half.
   b. Vocal cord mobility: Causes of fixed vocal cord are:
      i. Deep infiltration into muscle.
      ii. Large weight of growth mass.
      iii. Involvement of cricoarytenoid joint.
      iv. Subglottic extension.
      v. Invasion of recurrent laryngeal nerve.
   c. Extend of lesion: It may spread to vallecula, base of tongue, pyriform fossa.
3. Examination of neck—done for:
   a. Extralaryngeal spread:
      i. Growth of anterior commissure and subglottic region spread through cricothyroid membrane to produce midline swelling.
      ii. Invasion of thyroid cartilage and perichondritis which is painful and tender.
      iii. Invasion of thyroid gland and strap muscle.
   b. Nodule metastesis: Nodule for there size, member site, mobility and sides.

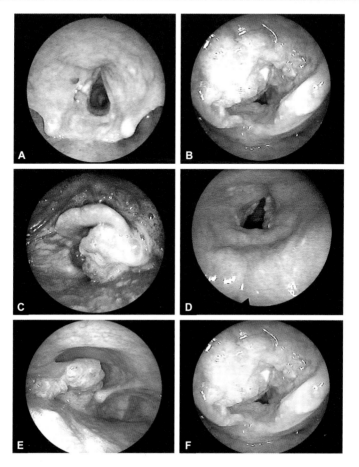

Figs 1 A to F: Presentation of different types of growth at different site in the larynx

Q.17 What are the various investigations done in cancer larynx?

Ans. 1. Routine blood investigation: HB, TLC, DLC, BT, CT, ESR.
2. Blood chemistry: Sugar, urea, critenine.
3. VDRL
4. Urine
5. Radiological: X-ray soft tissue neck and X-ray chest PA view.
6. CT scan and MRI.
7. Direct laryngoscopy.
8. Microlaryngoscopy.
9. Endoscopy (Fig. 2): For the growth.
10. Biopsy.

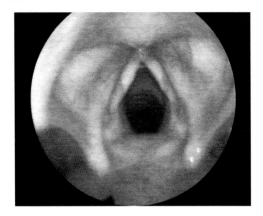

Fig. 2: Endoscopic view of normal larynx

Q.18 What are the finding in X-ray of soft tissue neck in cancer larynx?
Ans. Soft tissue neck lateral view shows:
1. Extent of lesion of epiglottis, ary epiglottic folds, arytenoids.
2. Involvement of pre-epiglottic space.
3. Destruction of thyroid cartilage.

Q.19 Why is important of CT scan in cancer larynx?
Ans. It is very useful for following reasons:
1. Find the extent of tumor.
2. Invasion of pre-epiglottic space or para-epiglottic spaces.
3. Destruction of cartilage.
4. Involvement of lymph node.
   It is also used in establishing the stage of diagnostic, therapeutic (line of deciding treatment) and prognostic importance.

Q.20 What is the importance of microlaryngoscopy in cancer larynx?
Ans. It is used in small lesion of vocal cord for:
1. Better visualization of the tumor.
2. To take, more accurate biopsy tissue in precise manner.

Q.21 What is the importance of supravital staining and biopsy in cancer larynx?
Ans. Toludine blue is applied to laryngeal lesion and than washed with saline and examined under the operating microscope. Carcinoma in situ and superficial carcinomas take up the white leukolplakia does not thus it select the area for biopsy.

Q.22 What is the importance of direct laryngoscopy in cancer larynx?
Ans. It is performed for the following reasons:
1. To direct the hidden areas of larynx.
2. To see the extent of disease.
3. To take the biopsy.

Q.23 What are the various hidden areas of the larynx which are not visible on mirror examination?

Ans. Hidden areas of the larynx are infrahyoid epiglottis, anterior commissure, subglottic area and ventricles.

Q.24 In which laryngeal cancer, the pre-epiglottic space is commonly involved?

Ans. Almost all growth of the supraglottic region invade the pre-epiglottic space but vocal cord cancer involves in later course of the disease in few cases.

Q.25 How does the glottic cancer present?

Ans. It presents as two distinct types:
1. A small tumor limited to the vocal cord.
2. A large tumor involving the glottic, supraglottic and subglottic, so it is called transglottic tumor.

Q.26 What are other pecularities of transglottic metastasis?

Ans. 1. It has high incidence of lymph node metastasis.
2. It spreads to the strap muscle (5%).
3. It spreads to thyroid gland (10%).

Q.27 What is the treatment of cancer larynx?

Ans. Treatment depends on the site of lesion, extent of lesion, presence or absence of node and distant metastasis. Treatment consists of:
1. Radiotherapy
2. Surgery:
   a. Conservation laryngeal surgery.
   b. Total laryngectomy.
   c. Radical neck dissection.
3. Chemotherapy
4. Combined therapy.

Q.28 What are disadvantages of laryngectomy in cancer larynx?

Ans. The disadvantages are: Loss of speech, anosmia, problem in lifting heavy weight, coughing and defecation.

Q.29 What are the advantages of laryngectomy?

Ans. 1. Response is good for larger tumor.
2. Full treatment at one sitting.

Q.30 What are advantages of radiotherapy?

Ans. 1. Preservation of speech and other laryngeal function.
2. Reduces the size of tumor.
3. Controls peripheral growth of tumor.
4. Useful in patients who is unfit or unwilling for surgery.

Q.31 What are the disadvantages of radiotherapy in cancer larynx?

Ans. The disadvantages are:
1. Not useful in large tumors.
2. High chances of flap necrosis in subsequent surgery.

3. Wound breakdown and fistula formation in subsequent surgery. Chances of initiation of malignancy at other normal site (second primary).

Q.32 What is the stagewise best treatment in cancer larynx?
Ans. Stage I: Radiotherapy.
Stage II: (a) Radiotherapy; (b) Radiotherapy or surgery.
Stage III: Surgery.
Stage IV: Combined modality.

Q.33 What are methods of communication in laryngectomized patients?
Ans. Methods of communication in laryngectomized patients are as follows:
1. Written language (pen and paper)
2. Aphonic lip speech (by trapping air in buccal cavity often combined with sign language)
3. Esophageal speech
4. Electrolarynx
5. Transoral pneumatic device
6. Tracheoesophageal speech
7. Blom-Singer's prosthesis
8. Panje prosthesis.

Q.34 Which type of growth carry a better prognosis in supraglottic cancer?
Ans. The prognosis of cauliflower-like growths is better than that of ulcerative growths.

Q.35 What are the factors which can affect the line of therapy?
Ans. These are:
1. Stage of growth
2. Histopathology
3. General fitness of the patient
4. Facilities available
5. Occupation: Profession with speech

Q.36 What is the treatment of glottic carcinoma?
Ans. 1. Carcinoma in situ: Treatment of transoral endoscopic CO_2 laser or stripping of vocal cord under microscope or radiotherapy, if invasive carcinoma on biopsy.
2. T1—carcinoma radiotherapy (if patient refused excision laser or laryngofissure).
3. T1—carcinoma with extension to anterior commissure: Radiotherapy or (frontolateral partial laryngectomy).
4. Ti—carcinoma with extension to arytenoids: Radiotherapy or conservation laryngeal surgery.
5. T2N0: With mobile cord radiotherapy
T2N0: With fixed cord-surgery
T3: Total laryngectomy
T4: Total laryngectomy.

Q.37 What is the treatment of subglottic carcinoma?
Ans. 1. T1and T2: Radiotherapy.
  2. T3 and T4: Total laryngectomy and postoperative radiotherapy.

Q.38 What factors should be considered in selecting the line of treatment in supraglottic cancer?
Ans. Following factors should be considered:
  1. Status of cervical lymph nodes.
  2. Mobility of cord.
  3. Age of patient.
  4. Status of lung function.
  5. Cartilage invasion.
  6. Subsites of supraglottic growth.
  7. Status of pre-epiglottic space involvement.
    – T1: Radiotherapy or CO_2 laser
    – T2: Supraglottic laryngectomy with or with RND or radiotherapy
    – T3: Total laryngectomy with RND + postoperative radiotherapy
    – T4: Total laryngectomy with RND+ postoperative radiotherapy.

Q.39 What should be the line of treatment for T2N0 glottic cancer?
Ans.

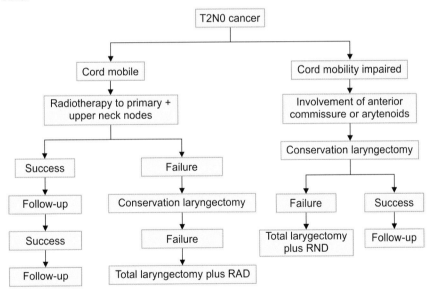

Q.40 What are the various methods of rehabilitation after total laryngectomy?
Ans. Methods of communication in laryngectomy patient are:
  1. Written language (paper and pen)
  2. Aphonic lip-speech with sign language.
  3. Esophageal speech.
  4. Electrolarynx.
  5. Transoral pneumatic device.

    6. Tracheoesophaged speech.
      – Blom–Singer prosthesis.
      – Panje prosthesis.

Q.41 What are the prognosis of radiotherapy in cancer larynx?

Ans. 1. Early lesion without involvement of cord mobility (90%).
    2. Superficial exophytic lesions of tip of epiglottis and aryepiglottic fold (70–90% cure rate).

Malignancy Pyriform Fossa

CASE: A 45-year-old man presented with increasing pain on swallowing for last 4 month with appearance of lump in right side of the upper neck for last 3 month. Examination of his neck reveals a neck lymph node in the right upper jugular group which is firm, nontender about 3 cm in diameter and mobile. Indirect laryngoscopy reveals an exophytic growth of the pyriform fossa, involving the lateral surface of aryepiglottic space.

Provisional Diagnosis: Malignancy Pyriform Fossa

Q.1 What is pyriform fossa?
Ans. It lies on either side of the larynx extend from pharyngoepiglottic fold to the upper end of the esophagus. It is bounded laterally by the thyrohyoid membrane and thyroid cartilage and medially by aryepiglottic fold, posterolateral surface of arytenoids and cricoids cartilages.

Q.2 What are the characteristic features of pyriform fossa?
Ans. 1. Richly supplied by lymphatics.
  2. Lymphatic drains to deep cervical chain in level IV and level VI after exit through thyrohyoid membrane.
  3. It is lined by squamous epithelium so almost all malignant lesions are squamous cell carcinoma.

Q.3 What is the extension and area of posterior pharyngeal wall?
Ans. It extends from the level of hyoid bone to the level of cricoarytenoids joint.

Q.4 What are the features of carcinoma pyriform fossa?
Ans. 1. It constitutes about 60% of all hypopharyngeal cancer.
  2. Common in male above 40 years.
  3. Growth remains asymptomatic for a long time because of large size fossa.
  4. Growth may be exophytic (Fig. 1B) or ulcerative (Fig. 1A) or deeply infiltrative.

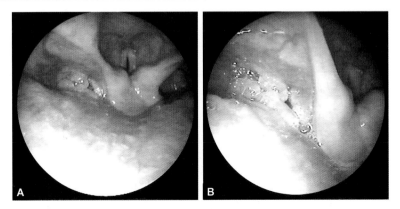

Figs 1A and B: Growth pyriform fossa

Q.5 What are the signs and symptoms of carcinoma pyriform fossa?

Ans. 1. Pricking sensation on swallowing—earliest symptoms.
2. Referred otalgia.
3. Pain on swallowing.
4. Increasing dysphagia.
5. Mass in the neck—may be first sign.
6. Hoarseness—indicates laryngeal involvement.
7. Stridor—due to laryngeal edema or spread of disease to larynx.

Q.6 How does the cancer pyriform fossa spread?

Ans. 1. Local spread: Upward to pharyngoepiglottic fold, valleculla and base of tongue, laterally it spreads to involve the:
   i. Thyroid cartilage: Thyrohyoid membrane, also involves thyroid gland.
   ii. Medially: It may involve aryepiglottic fold, paraglottic space and causes fixation of ipsilateral hemilarynx. It can also spread to pre-epiglottis space.
   iii. Posterior: It can extend to postcricoid region.
2. Lymphatic spread: Lymph node metastasis presents in 70% of cases at the time of presentation and about 35% has bilateral. Upper and middle group of jugular nodes are usually involved.
3. Hematogenous spread: Usually late and present in lung, liver and bones.

Q.7 What are the diagnostic investigations for cancer pyriform fossa?

Ans. 1. Indirect laryngoscopy and neck examination.
2. Barium swallow.
3. CT scan for extent of growth and status of lymph node.
4. Endoscopic examination for accurate assessment of growth and biopsy.

Q.8 What are the sites of origin for pyriform fossa cancer?

Ans. Tumor can arise from the lateral wall or the medial wall (marginal zone), or the apex.

Q.9 What are the levels for involving lymph node in pyriform fossa cancer?
Ans. Level II, III, IV and VI (rare).

Q.10 What is the treatment of pyriform fossa cancer?
Ans. 1. Early lesion: Radiotherapy.
  2. Growth limited to pyriform fossa not involving postcricoid.
    Treated:
    a. By total laryngectomy and partial pharyngectomy with primary closure of pharynx.
    b. With elective or prophylactic RND.
  3. Growth extending to postcricoid region: Treatment is total laryngectomy, pharyngectomy with block dissection neck.
    – Reconstruction of pharyngoesophageal segment with myocutaneous flaps or stomach pull-up.
    – Postoperative radiotherapy.

Postcricoid Carcinoma

CASE: A 30-year-old female presents with progressive painless persistent dysphagia with solids. There was no history of ear ache, change in voice and neck swelling. On neck examination, laryngeal crepitus was absent. Indirect laryngoscopy reveals exophytic growth visible posterior to larynx (Fig. 1) and with pooling of saliva in the pyriform fossa. Neck nodes were not palpable.

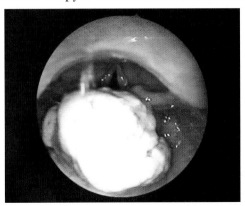

Fig. 1: Growth postcricoid region overshadow the posterior part of larynx

Provisional Diagnosis: Postcricoid Carcinoma

Q.1 What is postcricoid region?

Ans. It is an area between upper and lower borders of cricoid lamina. It is a part of anterior wall of laryngopharynx.

Q.2 What is postcricoid carcinoma?

Ans. Postcricoid region is one of the site of hypopharynx, the other regions are pyriform fossa and posterior pharyngeal wall. The development of carcinoma in postcricoid region has several features which are associated for site and its etiology. This region constitutes about 30% of laryngopharyngeal malignancies.

Q.3 What is significance of pain or otalgia in hypopharyngeal malignancies?

Ans. Pain and otalgia indicate growth of pyriform fossa or any other subsite growth extending to pyriform fossa and posterior pharyngeal wall.

Q.4 What is the significance of hoarseness of voice in hypopharyngeal carcinoma?

Ans. 1. Hoarseness of voice in pyriform fossa indicates laryngeal edema or spread of disease to larynx.
   2. Voice change may occur due to infiltration of recurrent laryngeal nerve or posterior cricoarytenoid muscles affecting vocal cord mobility in postcricoid carcinoma.

Q.5 What is the significance of hemoptysis?

Ans. It is unusual and present in pyriform fossa or posterior pharyngeal wall carcinoma.

Q.6 What are etiological factors for postcricoid carcinoma?

Ans. 1. Anemia.
   2. Plummer-Vinson syndrome (characterized by hypochromic microcytic anaemia), 1/3 of patient has PV syndrome.
   3. Alcohol and tobacco.
   4. Previous irradiation in neck.

Q.7 How does postcricoid carcinoma spread?

Ans. 1. Local spread occurs in annular fashion.
   2. Spreads mucosally.
   3. Invades cervical esophagus, arytenoids, trachea, thyroid gland and anterior mediastinum.
   4. Recurrent laryngeal nerve at cricoarytenoid joint.
   5. By lymphatic spread (20%) to paratrachial, medistinal and lower deep cervical nodes.
   6. Bilateral lymph node (5%).

Q.8 What are clinical features of postcricoid carcinoma?

Ans. 1. Common in female.
   2. Common between 20–30 years.
   3. Main presenting symptoms is progressive dysphasia.
   4. Other symptoms are progressive malnutrition and weight loss.
   5. Voice change—affecting larynx or its nerve.
   6. Indirect laryngoscopy: Variable
      a. Growth may not be visible.
      b. Pooling of secretion in hypopharynx.
      c. Edema and erythema of postcricoid region.
   7. Laryngeal crepitus: Absent (Bocca's sign).

Q.9 What is Chevalier Jackson's sign?

Ans. Pooling of saliva in pyriform fossa: Which is suggestive of underlying postcricoid growth.

Q.10 What are the investigations required?

Ans. 1. Blood for HB: Evidence of anemia.
2. X-ray soft tissue neck: Lateral view.
3. Barium swallow: To detect the lower extent of growth.
4. Endoscopy: For biopsy and to assess extent of growth.

Q.11 What is importance of barium swallow in postcricoid malignancy?

Ans. It provides following information
1. Assessment of tumor length.
2. Presence of any synchronous primary tumor of the esophagus.
3. Ascertain presence or absence of aspiration.
4. Assesses tumor mobility on vertebral column during deglutition.

Q.12 What is role of CT scan or MRI?

Ans. Useful in postirradiation neck.

Q.13 What is role of RND surgery in postcricoid malignancy?

Ans. Neck dissection is done when lymph node metastasis is present at level II, III, IV and VI.

Q.14 What is treatment of postcricoid carcinoma?

Ans. 1. Radiotherapy.
2. Laryngopharyngo-esophagectomy with stomach pull-up or in cases with failure radiotherapy for T3, T4 tumor.
3. Pharyngolaryngectomy with free jejunal transfer for T1, T2.

Q.15 What is TNM classification for hypopharynx cancer?

Ans. T–   Primary tumor, TX primary—can not be detected.
T0–   No evidence of primary tumor, Tis—carcinoma in situ.
T1–   Tumor limited to one sub site of hypopharynx and 2 cm or less in greatest dimension.
T2–   Tumor invades more than one sub site of hypopharynx or an adjacent site or measures >2 cm <4 cm in greatest diameter. Without fixation of hemilarynx.
T3–   Tumor measures >4 cm in greatest diameter or with hemilarynx fixation.
T4–   Tumor invades adjacent structures, thyroid cartilage, cricoid cartilage, carotid artery and soft tissues of neck, prevertebral muscle, fascia, thyroid gland, or esophagus.

SECTION 4

Diseases of the
Nose and Sinuses

Rhinophyma

CASE: Patient presents with multinodular firm mass with marked fissures and nodular surface on the nasal tip and adjuring dorsum (Fig. 1).

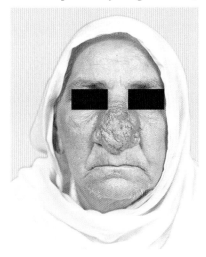

Fig. 1: Rhinophyma

Provisional Diagnosis: Rhinophyma

Q.1 What is rhinophyma?
Ans. It is an enormous progressive benign hypertrophy and hyperplasia of pilosebaceous glands as well as connective tissue at the tip of the nose. It is common in males by about 12 times.

Q.2 Who coined the term rhinophyma?
Ans. The term 'rhinophyma' is derived from the Greek word rhis (nose) and phyma (growth). The term was coined by Von Hebra.

Q.3 What are other names for it?
Ans. It is also called whisky nose, nodular nose, tomato nose, potato nose, hanging nose, elephantiasis nose, bulbous nose, cystadenofibroma of the nose, strawberry nose, hammer nose, double nose, rhino-blossum.

Q.4 What are predisposing factors ?

Ans. 1. Gastrointestinal disturbance.
2. Hormonal imbalance
3. Chronic inflammatory reaction may be produced by accumulation of large quantity of sebum in the dilated glands.

Q.5 What is pathogenesis of rhinophyma ?

Ans. It is considered to be final stage of acne rosacea. Early in the disease the dilation of blood vessels with increase in blood supply, causes overproduction of connective tissue which forms lobulated masses of variable size (from a pea to a cherry) being separated from one another by dense fibrous septum. It develops slowly in 5–20 years.

Q.6 What are the types on histological grounds?

Ans. Two forms:
1. Glandular form: Pilosebaceous glands increase in size and number.
2. Fibrotelangiectatic form: Proliferation of connective tissue predominates.

Q.7 What are clinical symptoms?

Ans. 1. Cosmetic deformity: Produced by nodular swelling at the nasal tip.
2. Nasal obstruction: In very large lesion.
3. Foul odors: Due to acumulation of sebum in between the lobules.

Q.8 What are clinical features of rhinophyma?

Ans. Clinically two verieties:
1. Smooth hypertrophic bulbous type: Seeped by sebaceous secretion and covered by telangiectatic blood vessel, giving it dusty red or purple color.
2. Multilobular tumor mass: Marked with fissures and nodulation, it is firm and has no sign of inflammation. Nasal rim and columela are not affected.

Q.9 What are complications or sequelae?

Ans. 1. Chances of malignancy change is about 10–15%.
2. Very big grotesque mass hung on nose.
3. Involvement and destruction of cartilage.

Q.10 What is treatment?

Ans. Main goal is to completely remove the lesion and restore the nasal contour without exposing nasal cartilage and bone and to avoid excess bleeding.
1. Surgical decortications.
2. Electrosurgical decortications.
3. Dermabrasion.
4. Excision with thick split thickness skin grafting.
5. Laser surgery.
6. Radiofrequency surgery.

CASE

50

Rhinolith

CASE: A child of 14 years presents with unilateral nasal obstruction with foul smelling discharge. Nasal examination reveals a gray brown or greenish-black mass with irregular surface (Figs 1A and B). On probing, gritting sensation with stone hard feel perceived. At places granulation tissues are present.

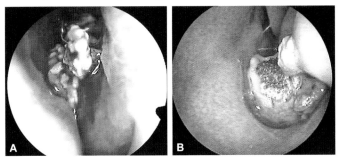

Figs 1A and B: Nasal endoscopy showing rhinolith

Provisional Diagnosis: Rhinolith

Q.1 What is rhinolith?

Ans. Stone formation in the nose due to slow deposition of calcium and magnesium salts around the nucleus of a small exogenous foreign body, clot or inspissated secretion. It grows into large, irregular stony mass filling the nasal cavity.

Q.2 What effects are produced by the stone?

Ans. Various effects are:
  1. May cause pressure necrosis of the septum (perforation of septum).
  2. May erode the lateral wall and enter the antrum (antrolith).
  3. Recurrent epistaxis.
  4. Neuralgic pain.
  5. Rarely may cause perforation of palate by pressure necrosis.

Q.3 What is characteristic of rhinolith?

Ans. It is often brittle and is liable to break into pieces while manipulations.

Q.4 What is treatment?

Ans. 1. Removal by intranasal route: Under general anesthesia.
  2. Lateral rhinotomy: In irregular and very large rhinolith.
  3. Endoscopic removal.

Q.5 What are differential diagnosis?

Ans. 1. FB nose.
  2. Polyp.
  3. Granuloma.
  4. Hypertrophic turbinate.

Antrochoanal Polyp
(Killian's Polyp)

CASE: A patient presents with nasal obstruction right side. Postnasal examination reveals a smooth pedunculated mass with faint yellowish tongue, at places semitranslucent, and at other place area is opaque (Figs 1 and 2). On nasal endoscopy same characteristic features are seen.

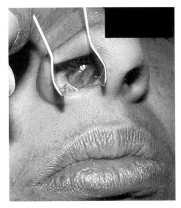

Fig. 1: Nasal polyp

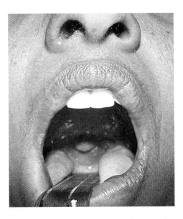

Fig. 2: Polyp hanging down in the oropharynx

Provisional Diagnosis: Antrochoanal Polyp

Q.1 What is a polyp?

Ans. Polyp is a non-neoplastic swelling which is actually a prolapsed edamatous respiratory mucosa. An antrochoanal polyp arises from the floor and medial wall of the antrum close to the accessory ostium, it enters the nasal cavity through its natural or accessory ostium and then passes backwards into the nasopharynx through the posterior choana. It also grows anteriorly to fill the nasal cavity, thus it is trilobular.

Q.2 Why does antrochoanal polyp passes into the posterior choana?

Ans. The choanal part is largest and antrochoanal polyp passes posteriorly due to the following reasons:
1. The direction of the opening of the maxillary ostia is downwards and backwards.
2. Direction of movement of cilia is towards nasopharynx.
3. Backward sloping of the floor the nasal cavity.
4. Inspiration creating a greater amount of negative pressure, pulls the polyp backwards.
5. Uncinate process direct the polyp posterior as emerges from the sinus.

Q.3 Which part of the antrochoanal polyp is smallest and what is its peculiarity?

Ans. Usually, the nasal part is smallest among the three parts. The tip of this part may show a discoloration (reddish or blackening) due to metaplasia of the exposed epithelium.

Q.4 What is etiology of antrochoanal polyp?

Ans. 1. It is uncommon (1% of polyps) and it is commonly seen in children, equally in both sexes. Predisposing factors are allergy and infection vasomotor, polysaccharide change, Bernoulli's phenomenon.
2. Polyp is covered by a pseudostratified columnar epithelium. The nasal part may show stratified squamous epithelium because of metaplastic changes. Eosinophils are found in plenty in the stroma.

Q.5 What are the clinical features?

Ans. 1. Nasal obstruction:
   – The classical presentation is good; inspiratory airway with blockage on expiration (result of the ball–valve effect of polyp blocking the posterior choana). Initially nasal obstruction is unilateral, but later on large size of polyp produces bilateral symptoms.
2. Mucoid discharge.
3. Snoring if large obstructing both choana.
4. Change in voice (hyponasality).
5. Conductivity deafness due to Eustachian tube obstruction.

Q.6 What are the findings on examination?

Ans. Polyp is mainly visible on the posterior choana, so postnasal mirror examination is must. Polyp looks like a smooth, grayish white, spherical mass, in the choana (Fig. 3). Later on when it grows in size, anteriorly can visible in the nasal cavity (Fig. 1). The polyp is soft, insensitive, nontender and does not bleed on probe examination.

Q.7 What are the findings in X-ray?

Ans. 1. X-ray PNS water's view shows an opaque maxilla antrum on affected side with a shadow on the nasal fossa (Fig. 4).

2. X-ray lateral view nasopharynx shows a swelling in the nasopharynx with a column of air above and behind the mass (Fig. 5). CT scan is required for confirmation of diagnosis.

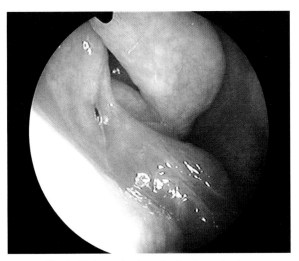

Fig. 3: Endoscopic view of antrochoanal polyp

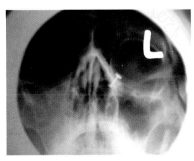

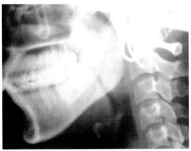

Fig. 4: X-ray PNS water 's view shows the right antrum hazy with obliteration of nasal airway

Fig. 5: X-ray nasopharynx (Lateral view) soft tissue shadow in the nasopharynx with air column above and behind (Crescent sign)

Q.8 **What is difference between the nasal component of polyp with antral component?**

Ans. Grossly, the nasal component of the polyp is similar to common nasal polyp in appearance while the maxillary antral component is thin fluid-filled cyst. A small fibrous band joins the two components as it passes out of the sinus.

Q.9 **What is the anatomical relation of antrochoanal polyp?**

Ans. The anatomical relation of antrochoanal polyp is as follows:
1. Maxillary sinus component with its attachment
2. Maxillary osteum
3. Ostiomeatal complex
4. Posterior choana
5. Nasopharynx
6. Anterior nasal components.

Q.10 **What are findings in CT scan in antrochoanal polyp?**

Ans. Mass occupying the maxillary antrum and extending into the nasopharynx is seen in different cuts. The attachment site in the antrum may be identified. In case of angiomatic polyp widening or destruction of ostium is seen.

Q.11 **What are various types of antrochoanal polyp?**

Ans. Depending on the basis of predominant stromal element sinonasal polyps are classified into five types: edematous, glandular, fibrosis, cystic and angiomatous or angioctatic polyp.

Q.12 **Describe differential diagnosis of antrochoanal polyp?**

Ans. It should be differentiated from juvenile nasopharyngeal angiofibroma, hemartoma, nasopharyngeal carcinoma, meningocoel, hypertrophic posterior turbinate, sphenochoanal polyp, nasopharyngeal rhinosporidiosis, Thornwaldt's cyst, craniopharyngioma.

Q.13 **What is treatment of antrochoanal polyp?**

Ans. 1. Transnasal/transoral polypectomy—before the 15 years of age (before the second molar tooth erupts).
2. Caldwell Luc's operation—was done frequently in the past. It is indicated in recurrent polyp or if endoscope is not available.
3. Endoscopic polypectomy (FESS)—with middle meatal antrostomy by joining the accessory and nasal ostia together, entire polyp is removed under direct vision. Microdebrider may be used to remove the entire polyp or antral part.

CASE

52

Ethmoidal Polypi

CASE: A patient presents with bilateral progressive nasal obstruction, sneezing and rhinorrhea of 6 months duration.

Multiple, grayish-white/bluish–white pedunculated smooth glistening masses in the both nose, coming out from ethmoidal area. Probe test shows soft, mobile, insensitive, non-fragile masses do not bleed on touch.

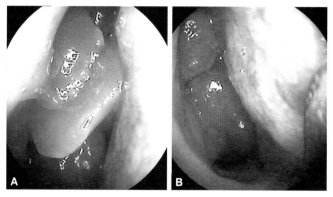

Figs 1A and B: Bilateral nasal polyposis presenting as multiple grape-like mass

Provisional Diagnosis: Ethmoidal Polypi

Q.1 What is diagnosis?

Ans. Bilateral ethmoidal polypi or nasal polyposis (Fig. 1).

Q.2 What are clinical signs for favoring diagnosis of ethmoidal polypi?

Ans. These are multiple, look like bunch of grapes, bilateral, seem to arise from anterior middle and posterior groups of ethmoidal cells.

Q.3 What else can be clinical findings?

Ans. 1. There may be associated infection (Pus) in the middle meatus. There may be mucinous nasal discharge in the nasal cavity. In long-standing cases, there may be expansion or broadening of the external nose, known as ''frog face'' due to large number of polypoidal masses trying to come out through anterior nares.

2. Some times the polypi may be reddish due to squamous metaplasia (due to exposure to irritants) in anterior most polyps.
3. Hyponasal voice (rhinolalia clausa) is present due to bilateral nasal obstruction.

Q.4 What are the causes of frog face deformity in ethmoidal polyps?
Ans. 1. Large number of ethmoidal polyps
2. Long standing multiple masses
3. Expansion of ethmoidal labyrinths.

Q.5 How the ethmoidal polypi are formed?
Ans. Inilially there is focal mucosal edema (due to extracellular fluid) in the ethmoidal sinuses. Due to their weight, gravity and excessive sneezing, they tend to enlarge and hungs downwards and finally become pedunculated. At this stage obstruction occurs in venous return due to kinking and twisting leading to more oedema.

Q.6 What are the main symptoms of nasal polyposis?
Ans. 1. Disease usually occurs in young adults and rare in children. Men are more frequently affected.
2. Main symptoms are progressive nasal obstruction (usually bilateral), nasal discharge and sneezing due to associated allergy.
3. There may be hyposmia or anosmia, postnasal drip and headache (vacuum headache). Sometimes excessive lacrimation may occur due to blockage of nasolacrimal duct.

Q.7 What are the complications of ethmoidal polypi?
Ans. Complications are:
1. Rhinosinusitis.
2. Ear infection
3. Hypertelorism or frog face deformity—as a late complication especially associated with fungal sinusitis.
4. Mucocele—due to obstruction of the sinus ostia.

Q.8 What investigations are required to confirm the diagnosis of ethmoidal polyps?
Ans. X-ray paranasal sinuses—in detecting the extent of the disease in the sinuses.
a. CT scan of paranasal sinuses (Fig. 2). It is the investigation of choice. It reveals the extent of the disease, the condition of lamina papyracea and also the posterior ethmoidal air cells and cribriform plate.
b. Biopsy—can be done in doubtful cases.
c. Nasal smear for eosinophils.
d. Blood for Hb, TLC, DLC, TEC, BTCT

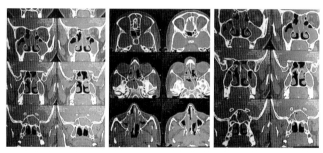

Fig. 2: CT scan: Sinonasal polyposis

Q.9 What are other conditions should be differentiated from nasal polyps?

Ans. It should be differentiated from hypertrophic turbinate, cystic middle turbinate, inverted papilloma, antrochoanal polyp, nasopharyngeal fibroma, granulomatous masses, fungal granuloma and other tumors.

Q.10 What is the criteria to differentiate between polyp and inferior turbinate?

Ans. Nasal polyp is pale or gray in color, insensitive and mobile on probing while the middle turbinate is pink, sensitive and immobile on probing.

Q.11 What is etiology of nasal polyposis?

Ans. Etiology of nasal polyposis is very complex and is not well understood. It is primarily disease of the ethmoidal sinuses from which the mucosal changes also extend to other sinuses, commonly the maxillary antrum followed by frontal sinuses and sphenoid sinuses.

The etiological factors that are possibly responsible are:
1. Allergy: In most cases allergy, asthma and nasal polypi are seen to co-exist and 90% cases have eosinophilia.
2. Infection: Chronic rhinosinusitis also found to be cause of nasal polyposis.
3. Bernoulli's phenomenon: When fluid/air passes through a constricted area at a high velocity there is a sudden drop of pressure distal to constriction thus resultant negative pressure sucks the mucosa of the sinuses in the nasal cavity.
4. Vasomotor imbalance: Also may be contributory factor.
5. Ciliary motility or abnormal composition of mucus.
6. Various other diseases may also be associated with it.

Q.12 What are other conditions may be associated with nasal polyposis?

Ans. Various other diseases may be associated with formation of nasal polyposis.
1. Cystic fibrosis: 20% of patients with cystic fibrosis have bilateral polyposis, specially occurring in children.

2. Samter's triad: Consists of nasal polypi, asthma and aspirin intolerance. 36% of the patients with aspirin intolerance may show polypi.
3. Allergic fungal sinusitis: Almost all cases have nasal polypi.
4. Kartagener's syndrome: Consists of bronchiectasis, sinusitis, sinus versus ciliary dyskinesia.
5. Young's syndrome: Sinopulmonary disease, azoospermia and nasal polypi.
6. Churg-Strauss syndrome: Consists of asthma, fever, eosinophilia, vasculitis and granuloma.
7. Nasal mastocytosis: Chronic nasal disease in which mucosa is infiltrated with mast cells with few eosinophils. Skin test for IgE level and allergy is normal.

Q.13 What are the histopathological features of ethmoidal polypi?
Ans. 1. Ciliated columnar lining epithelium with or without squamous metaplasia.
2. Fibrillar stroma with fluid-filled spaces in the submucosa, with numerous lymphocytes, eosinophils and plasma cells.
3. Scanty blood vessels and nerve fibers.

Q.14 What is the criteria for grading the polyp size?
Ans. Polyp size can be grade as:
Grade 1: Polyp is small in middle meatus and hidden or visible on endoscopy after retracting the middle turbinate medially.
Grade 2: Polyp is small in the middle meatus and hidden but just at the level of middle turbinate.
Grade 3: Polyp which just comes out of middle meatus. Polyp is directly visible on anterior rhinoscopy filling the nasal cavity.

Q.15 What are the common sites of origin of nasal polypi.
Ans. Multiple nasal polypi always arise from lateral wall, never from septum and floor of the nose. Common sites are middle meatus, ethmoidal labyrinth, uncinate process, bulla ethmoidalis, ostia of sinuses, medial surface and edge of middle turbinate.

Q.16 What is the treatment of nasal polyp?
Ans. 1. Anti-histaminics: Control allergy and early polypoidal change with edematous mucosa.
2. Steroids: Useful in:
   a. Early stage specially in those having asthma associated.
   b. To reduce the volume and size of polypi preoperatively.
   c. To prevent recurrence.
   d. Regression of disease where surgery is not possible.
   Mostly prednisolone (30–60 mg) for 4-7 days and then it is tapered for 1–3 weeks. Steroid appears to depend on the presence or absence of eosinophilia. Patient with polypi not dominated by eosinophil i.e. cystic fibrosis, primary ciliary dyskinesia or Young's syndrome may not respond to steroid.

3. Antibiotic: Can be given for bacterial superadded infection, roxythromycin or azithromycin is commonly used. Steroid nasal spray can be given for short period like budesonide, fluticasone, mometasone. These help in reducing the size of polyps.
4. Surgical treatment.

Q.17 What are the surgical procedures to deal with ethmoidal polypi?

Ans. 1. Intranasal polypectomy with ethmoidectomy: Intranasal all polypi are removed, the ethmoidal cells are uncapped. It is somewhat blind procedure and not completely safe, not done very commonly now.
2. External ethmoidectomy (Howarth's operation): Ethmoidal air cells are approached by external route through an incision medial to the inner canthus of the eye. This is also not done commonly now.
3. Transantral ethmoidectomy (Jansen-Horgan's operation): It is used to deal with polypi involving the maxillary antrum and also to approach the posterior ethmoidal air cell polypi through transantral route. It is done by a Caldwell–Luc approach.
4. Endoscopic sinus surgery (ESS or FESS) is better technique in which polyps are removed precisely as well as the clefts in the middle meatus are also opened. Thus, the chances of recurrence are less.
Ostia are widened; ventilation and drainage is established in all sinuses. The use of microdebrider has made the procedure safer and faster, providing precise tissue cutting and decreased hemostasis with better visualization.

Q.18 What are the complications of FESS in nasal polypi?

Ans. Complications of FESS in nasal polypi can be:
1. Bleeding.
2. Synechiae.
3. Diplopia.
4. Subcutaneous emphysema.
5. Blindness.
6. Closure of antrostomy.
7. Toothache.
8. Infection.
9. CSF leak.
10. Epiphora.

Q.19 Which anesthesia is better in surgery of ethmoidal polyps?

Ans. General anesthesia is better as:
1. Under LA the polyps shrink.
2. Recurrence is common in LA.
3. Excellent access.

Q.20 What are the special investigations required for childhood polyp?

Ans. Investigations required are:
1. Sweat test: Diagnostic test for cystic fibrosis.
2. Biopsy: To exclude tumors.

3. Fresh sample of nasal lining for special ciliary function test.
4. Electron microscopy.
5. To cheek the ciliary structure.
6. CT scan: To exclude meningocele.

Q.21 What is the advantage of nasal polypi surgery?

Ans. Removal of complete nasal polypi and sinuses disease, usually improves pulmonary system. There is relief in nasal obstruction and snoring. Olfaction (smell perception) returns. Normalization of quality of life activities like sleep, talking, chewing, food habits restored.

Deviated Nasal Septum

CASE: A young boy presented with right side nasal obstruction and producing projection like abnormality in the anterior nares (Caudal deviation) on left side. Examination reveals 'C' shaped deformity of nasal septum more on right side (Figs 1A and B).

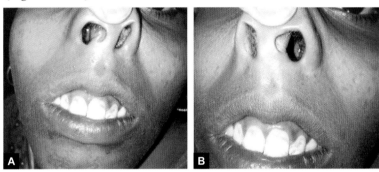

Figs 1A and B: DNS—right

Provisional Diagnosis: Deviated Nasal Septum

Q.1 What is the diagnosis?
Ans. Deviated nasal septum 'C' shaped with caudal deviation.

Q.2 What is deviated nasal septum (DNS)?
Ans. Nasal septum is a midline partition of the bone and cartilage covered with mucous membrane on either side dividing the nasal cavity into two, right and left. Deviation or deflection of part or whole of septum on the either side is called DNS.

Q.3 What are 'C' and 'S' shaped deviation?
Ans. 1. 'C' shaped deviation: Both the cartilage and bony septum is deviated to one side (Fig. 2).
  2. 'S' shaped deviation: The cartilaginous part is deviated to one side, whereas the bony part gets deviation to opposite side.

Q.4 What is the main point in favor of diagnosis?

Ans. Bilateral nasal obstruction with 'C' of Shaped deviation of the nasal septum with projection of anterior edge of nasal septum.

Q.5 What are causes of nasal obstruction?

Ans. The nasal obstruction can be unilateral or bilateral. The causes of unilateral nasal obstruction are:

1. 'C' shaped DNS (Fig. 2).
2. Hypertrophic turbinate or unilateral concha bullosa.
3. Foreign body (children).
4. Rhinolith.
5. Unilateral atrophic rhinitis.
6. Antrochoanal polyp.
7. Rhinosporidiosis.
8. Tumors of the nose and sinuses.

The causes of bilateral nasal obstruction are:

1. S-shaped DNS.
2. Rhinitis.
3. Chronic sinusitis.
4. Chronic hypertrophic rhinitis.
5. Atrophic rhinitis.
6. Vasomotor rhinitis.
7. Allergic rhinitis.
8. Ethmoidal polypi.
9. Hypertrophic adenoid.
10. Growth nasopharynx.

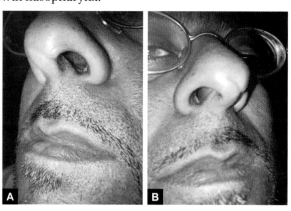

Figs 2A and B Caudal deviation

Q.6 What are other clinical variations and patterns of nasal obstruction?

Ans. Nasal obstruction can be intermittent, progressive, relieved with decongestant medication, or with steroid nasal spray, influenced by bath and washing face and sexual intercourse and drug-induced obstruction.

Causes of intermittent nasal obstruction are:
1. Allergic rhinitis.
2. Ethmoidal polypi.
3. Vasomotor rhinitis.

Causes of progressive nasal obstruction:
1. Polyp.
2. Malignancies.

Causes of nasal obstruction relieved by decongestant medications are:
1. Inflammatory.
2. Vasomotor rhinitis.
3. Polypi.

Nasal obstruction relieved by steroid spray are:
1. Allergic rhinitis.
2. Vasomotor rhinitis.
3. Chronic rhinitis.
4. Nasal polyposis.

Drug-induced nasal obstruction can be caused by:
1. Antihypertensives: Methyl dopa, guanethidine, reserpine, hydralazine, prazosin, etc.
2. Beta blockers: Propranolol and nadolol.
3. Antidepressants and tranquilizers: Thioridazine, librium, alprazolam.
4. Oral contraceptives.
5. Ergot alkaloids.
6. Antithyroid drugs.
7. Topical decongestants by rebound action.

Nasal obstruction can also occur after sexual intercourse: Honeymoon rhinitis.

Q.7 What is physiological classification of nasal obstruction?

Ans. 1. Nasal obstruction can occur during inspiration or during expiration.
2. The causes of nasal obstruction during inspiration: when obstruction in the anterior part of nostril, e.g. foreign body, nasal polyp, DNS, etc.
3. Nasal obstruction during expiration occurs mainly in antrochoanal polyp, here inspiration smoothly occurs but during expiration it blocks the choana (ball valve).

Q.8 What are etiological factors for DNS?

Ans. Common factors responsible for DNS are developmental, accidental trauma, natal trauma (forceps delivery), antenatal (abnormal posture), mouth breathers, cleft lip and palate, mass in nose, etc.

Q.9 What are common types of DNS?

Ans. Types are: (1) 'C' shaped, (2) 'S' shaped (Fig. 3), (3) Caudal deviation (Fig. 4), (4) Spur, (5) Thick septum (reduplication).

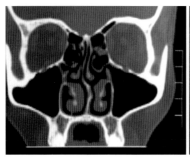 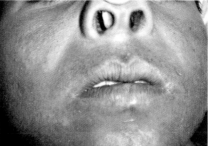

Fig. 3: CT scan: 'S' shaped DNS   **Fig. 4:** Caudal dislocation

Q.10 What is Cottle's classification of nasal septum?

Ans. Cottle's classification:

(i) Simple DNS, (ii) Obstructed DNS, (iii) Impacted.

1. Simple DNS: Mild deflection of the septum that obstructed the nasal cavity.
2. Obstructed DNS: Severe deflection of the septum which may touch the lateral wall of the nose but on applying decongestant, the turbinates shrink away from the septum.
3. Impacted DNS: Marked angulation of the septum that lies in contact with lateral wall even after application of vasoconstrictors.

Q.11 What is spur and caudal dislocation?

Ans. Spur is angulation at bony and cartilaginous junction of nasal septum. Caudal dislocation: Anterior end of the nasal septum bulges out of the nasal cavity on retraction of the nasal tip.

Q.12 What are other associated findings in the nose in deviated nasal septum?

Ans. 1. There is compensatory hypertrophy of the contralateral side in 'C' shaped DNS.
2. Presence of pus in middle meatus indicates sinusitis as complication of DNS.

Q.13 What are common symptoms of DNS?

Ans. 1. Nasal obstruction: Usually unilateral which later becomes bilateral due to turbinate hypertrophy, resulting in mouth breathing.
2. Headache: May occur due to sinusitis or pressure by deviation on the lateral wall.
3. Anterior ethmoidal nerve syndrome: By impacted deviated nasal septum impinging on the area of anterior ethmoidal nerve over the middle and inferior turbinate, causing pain in an area from super-ciliary ridge over the nasal bones to nasal tip.
4. Snoring.
5. Hyposmia or anosmia.
6. Fullness of the ears, decreased hearing due to Eustachian tube block.

7. Deformity of the nose.
8. Epistaxis: Occurs due to drying effects of air currents that impinges upon vessels stretched over the spur, causing rupture of vessel wall.

Q.14. Describe pathophysiology of DNS.

Ans. Mild DNS do not produce any symptoms.

In case of gross deviation, the opposite concave side becomes roomy, so more air enter through it. The inferior turbinate on wider side get compensatory hypertrophy in order to maintain the physiological function of warming and humidification. Thus, it results in sense of obstruction on this side also (Paradoxical obstruction).

Deviated septum may cause obstruction of sinus ostia, leading to stagnation of secretion which results in sinusitis. The infection spreads mucosal continuity and may cause edema of the mucosa of the Eustachian tube which may result in secretory otitis media.

Q.15 What is Cottle's areas of the nasal cavity?

Ans. The nasal cavity area is divided into five areas according to site of obstruction or pathology, i.e. vestibular, valvular, attic, turbinal or choanal.

Q.16. What investigations are to be done?

Ans. A diagnosis is always made on clinical ground. However, certain investigations can be done to exclude other complications or coexisting diseases.

1. X-ray PNS (Water's views): May not always show the site and degree of obstruction.
2. CT scan: Helpful in showing site and degree of obstruction and associated other abnormalities.

Q.17 What is the treatment of deviated nasal septum?

Ans. No treatment is required in asymptomatic DNS.

Symptomatic DNS should be corrected by surgery.

The indications are:

1. DNS with persistent unilateral nasal obstruction.
2. DNS causing sinusitis and epistaxis.
3. DNS with snoring.
4. DNS with caudal dislocation.
5. DNS with external nasal deformity.

Two types of operation done are:

a. Septoplasty.
b. Submucous resection (SMR).

Q.18 What is SMR?

Ans. It is an operation in which much of deviated cartilaginous and bony septum is removed by the submucosal dissection leaving the dorsal and caudal struts of cartilage intact in order to prevent deformity of the external nose.

Q.19 What is the septoplasty?

Ans. 1. It is an operation is which only the deviated portion of the septum is removed and the rest of the septum framework is retained.

2. It is indicated in cartilaginous deviation. It can be done in children and young females.

Q.20 What are contraindications of SMR?

Ans. It should not be done in children or young females.

1. In children, surgery on bony framework of midface may interfare with growth of the nose resulting in deformity.

2. In young female, surgery is not performed because of fear of cosmetic disfigurement.

Q.21 What are complications of SMR operation.

Ans. Complications are:

1. Septal hematomas.
2. Septal abscess.
3. Septal perforation.
4. Flapping septum.
5. Drooping of the tip.
6. Saddle nose.

Q.22 What are other indications for SMR operation.

Ans. 1. As an approach to transseptal vidian neurectomy.

2. As an approach for pituitary surgery.

3. To obtain a cartilage graft material for reconstructive surgery.

Q.23 What are differences between septoplasty and SMR operation?

Ans. 1. SMR is usually indicated for deviations posterior to the vertical line passing between the nasal process of frontal and maxillary bones (Cottle's line) while septoplasty for anterior segment deviations.

2. In SMR, Killian's incision is used while in septoplasty, Freer's hemitransfixation incision is used.

3. Mucoperichondrium is elevated on both side in SMR while it is mostly elevated on one side in septoplasty.

4. In SMR, both cartilage and bone are removed leaving the dorsal and caudal struts of cartilage while in septoplasty only deviated part of cartilage is removed after making it free from its only attachments and then it is repositioned after suitable scoring.

5. Complications are common in SMR but rare in septoplasty.

6. Revision surgery is difficult in SMR but can be possible in septoplasty.

7. Chance of redeviation is less in SMR while more chance of redeviation in septoplasty.

Q.24 What is endoscopic septoplasty?

Ans. Nasal endoscopy allows precise preoperative identification of septal pathology and its associated lateral nasal wall abnormalities and help in better planning of endoscope aided septal surgery. It fulfils almost all criteria of an ideal septal surgery by providing good visualization, with adequate illumination, and exact evaluation of the pathology and only essentially required manipulation and resection, preventing over exposure of the septal framework thus reducing the scope for a revision surgery.

Q.25 **What are ideal criteria for surgical correction of the nasal septum?**
Ans. Ideal criteria (Nayak et al. 1998) are:
1. Should relieve the nasal obstruction.
2. Should be conservative.
3. Should not produce iatrogenic deformity.
4. Should not compromise the osteomeatal complex.
5. Should relieve all the contact areas.
6. Must have the scope for a revision surgery, if required later.

54 Osteomyelitis of the Nasal Bone

CASE: There is an sinus on the nose having sprouting granulation tissue and thick purulent discharge, it is fixed to bone. At one place colored bone is visible with irregular surface, bone is tender, surrounding skin is inflamed.

Provisional Diagnosis: Osteomyelitis

Q.1 What is diagnosis?
Ans. Possible diagnosis: Chronic osteomyelitis.

Q.2 What is chronic osteomyelitis?
Ans. It is an infection of bone which becomes chronic due to ineffective treatment leading either to formation of dead bone or formation of an abscess.

Q.3 What are the causes of osteomyelitis?
Ans. Causes are:
　　1. Sequele of acute osteomyelitis.
　　2. Following trauma or operation on bone.
　　3. Brodie's abscess.

Q.4 What is sequestrum?
Ans. It is dead piece of the bone in osteomylitic cavity either separated or in the process of separation.

Q.5 How sequestrum is formed in osteomyelitis cavity?
Ans. Initially an abscess forms in subperiosteal area and then comes into bony canal. Vessels undergo infective thrombosis, ischemia of bone result into necrosis, dead bone and ultimately separated from living bone in the osteomyelitis cavity.
　　New subperiosteal bone is formed in osteomyelitis cavity to strengthen the bone is called involucrum.

Q.6 What are different type of sequestrum?
Ans. According to character, these are:
　　1. Feathery—tubercular.
　　2. Ivory—syphilis.
　　3. Colored—subcutaneous bone.

Q.7 What is colored sequestrum?

Ans. If sequestrum is formed in subcutaneous bone like of the nose, maxilla or zygoma which are exposed to air. Iron from the broken down hemoglobin reacts with hydrogen-sulfide of the air and forms iron sulfide. This is deposited on the exposed surface of the bone which becomes black in color.

Q.8 Why is one surface of sequestrum rough, irregular while the other surface is smooth?

Ans. One surface is smooth as it is in contact with cavity and other surface is rough because it is covered with granulation tissue.

Q.9 Clinical features of sequestrum formation.

Ans. Sprouting granulation tissue at the mouth of sinus is indication of formation of sequestrum.

Q.10 What are investigations required?

Ans. 1. X-ray of local part
2. Pus for culture and sensitivity.
3. CT scan.

Q.11 What are the findings in X-ray?

Ans. 1. Dense white bone in the bony cavity.
2. Involucrum and opening may be visible.
3. Patchy sclerosis around the cavity.

Q.12 What are differential diagnosis of chronic osteomyelitis ?

Ans. Chronic osteomyelitis.
1. Tubercular osteomyelitis.
2. Soft tissue infection.
3. Bony tumor.
4. Fungal infection.

Q.13 What is the treatment of osteomyelitis?

Ans. Surgery is definite treatment, antibiotic can only control acute exacerbation.

Q.14 What is the aim of surgical treatment?

Ans. Aims are:
1. Removal of dead bone.
2. Removal of pus and granulation tissue from the cavity.
3. Obliteration of the cavity by removal of ridge of bone from walls on both side (saucerization).

Q.15 What are complications of osteomyelitis?

Ans. These are:
1. Pathological fracture at the weak point.
2. Amyloidosis.
3. Squamous cell carcinoma at sinus tract.
4. Growth abnormality as growth plate or center is involved.

CASE

55

Atrophic Rhinitis

CASE: A 30-year-old female presents with history of nasal obstruction, loss of smell perception and scanty nasal discharge with profuse crust for about 10 years. On anterior rhinoscopy nasal cavity is roomy, filled with purulent nasal discharge and greenish foul smelling crusts in the roof, lateral wall (Fig. 1A) and septum. The mucosa was atrophic, dry and reddish. Turbinates are grossly atrophic, reduced in size, the mucosa was insensitive on probing. Posterior rhinoscopy revealed dryness of mucosa with a few crust in the choana (Fig. 1B). Examination of throat showed dryness of mucosa.

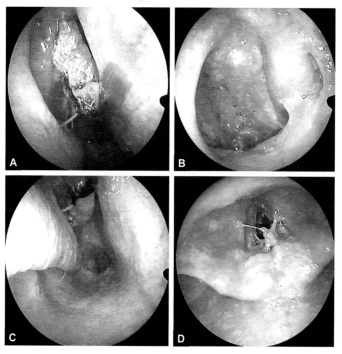

Figs 1A to D: (A) Middle turbinate and crusts; (B) Crusts in the nasopharynx; (C) Roomy nasal cavity (note that nasopharynx is seen); (D) Atrophic laryngitis crusts are also seen in subglottis

Provisional Diagnosis: Atrophic Rhinitis

Q.1 What is atrophic rhinitis?

Ans. Atrophic rhinitis is a chronic inflammatory disease of nose, characterized by progressive atrophy of the nasal mucosa and underlying turbinate bones, resulting in a roomy nasal cavity (Fig. 1C) and yellowish green crusting with foul smell. It is also called ozoena.

Q.2 What are various other type of atrophic rhinitis?

Ans. Atrophic rhinitis is usually classified into two types:
1. Primary atrophic rhinitis.
2. Secondary atrophic rhinitis which is secondary to trauma and (major nasal surgery), irradiation, or chronic nasal infection (tuberculosis, leprosy, scleroma, syphilis) and other granulomatous disease (midline Stewart's granuloma, sarcoidosis, fungal granuloma).

Q.3 What is its geographical distribution?

Ans. It is common in India, China, Pakistan, Bangladesh, and Egypt. It is uncommon in Europe, North America and other developed countries.

Q.4 What are etiological factors in atrophic rhinitis?

Ans. The exact etiology is not known, but the various contributory factors are (Mnemonic HERNIA):
1. Age: Often at puberty, common between 15–40 years.
2. Sex: More common in female.
3. Heredity: It may occur in members of the same family.
4. Autoimmune: Altered reactivity of immune mechanism causing destruction of mucosa, neurovascular and granular elements decrease in absolute number of T-lymphocytes.
5. Endocrinal dysfunction: Imbalance of sex hormones more common in female, at puberty age; it is common after menopause.
6. Nutritional: Iron, zinc, vitamin A, may contribute.
7. Infection: Bacterial infection by *Coccobacillus* to foetidus ozenae, *Klebsiella ozaezane, Bacillus mucosus*, and diphtheroids may be causative or secondary factors.
8. Mechanical theory of Zaufal:
   a. Skeletal defect (roomy nasal cavity due to gross DNS to one side) may cause unilateral atrophic rhinitis on the roomy side.
   b. Broad nose due to spacious (widnes) in side nose causing dryness of mucosa by a strong blast of air in the nose.
9. Reflex sympathetic dystrophy syndrome: Air-flow falling directly on the lateral wall initial artificial synapse between afferent somatic nerve and efferent sympathetic fibers. That causes initial hyperemia followed by obterative (vasculitis).
10. Past history of infectious fever found in most cases, like smallpox, chickenpox, kala-azar, etc.
11. Suppuration of nose and sinus: Past history of chronic and recurrent rhinites may damage to mucosa and glands.

12. Blood group: More common in blood group 'A' and 'B'.
13. Immunological factors.
14. AIDS: More common in AIDS patients.
15. Surfactant deficiency: Change in phospholipid prefile in nasal aspirate.

Q.5 What are pathological features of atrophic rhinitis?

Ans. 1. Complete metaplasia of columnar ciliated epithelium into stratified squamous epithlium with hyperkeratosis and crust formation. There is atrophy of cilia due to ischemic atrophy with pale mucosa.
2. Basement membrane is intact and thick.
3. Mucous glands and serous glands become scanty, indistinct in outline with smaller lumen (atrophic).
4. Deposition of collagen tissue in submucous area (fibrosis of lamina propria).
5. Atrophy changes in the bone, there may be fragmentation (absorption of bone).
6. Atrophy of nerve, loss of sensation so patient feels obstruction.
7. Venous spaces are atrophied.
8. Atrophy of olfactory nerve: Loss of smell.
9. Terminal arterials (in type I) show endarteritis and periarteritis. There may be perivascular fibrosis in form of cuffing. In type II, there may be vasodilation.
10. Paranasal sinuses are small due to arrested development.
11. The lamina or tunica propria: An abundant round cell infiltration, with occasional mast cells.

Q.6 What are peculiarities of symptoms of atrophic rhinitis?

Ans. 1. Nasal obstruction may true due to crusting block or may be false. Nasal cavity is roomy still patient may complaint of obstruction even in the absence of crust which is due to nonfeeling of air passing through the nose (loss of sensation due to nerve atrophy).
2. Epistaxis may occur on separation of crusts.
3. Crusting: Foul smell crusts comes out the nose periodically.
4. Anosmia (merciful anosmia): Patient cannot smell the foul smell of his own crust of the nose.
5. Foul smelling: There is foul smell, which keeps away the relatives of patient causing social problem.
6. Dryness of the nose and some time of the pharynx.
7. Diminished hearing due to blockage of Eustachian tube by the crust.
8. A constant desire to clear the throat.
9. Discomfort in throat due to crust trickling down in throat.

Q.7 What are diagnostic findings in atrophic rhinitis?

Ans. 1. External nose: The bridge of the nose may sometime depressed due to atrophy of the nasal septum.
2. Anterior rhinostomy:
   – Mucosa—pale and atrophic, covered with grayish or greenish foul smelling crusts

- Turbinates—are atrophic, leading to roomy nose so nasopharynx is directly visible
- Nasal septum—may occasionally have perforation
- Disease is usually bilateral but may be unilateral
- Loss of sensation—due to atrophy of trigeminal nerve endings
3. Posterior rhinoscopy: Crusting are seen, mucosa is dry and atrophic.
4. Crusting at orifice of Eustachian tube may cause sign of retraction of drum or middle-ear effusion.
5. Examination of larynx: Dry glazy and inflamed mucosa.

Q.8 What are the complications of atrophic rhinitis?

Ans. 1. Atrophic pharyngitis.
2. Atrophic laryngitis (Fig. 1D).
3. Maggots nose due to foul smell and loss of sensation.
4. Sinusitis.
5. Middle-ear infection blockage of Eustachian tube opening by crust, spread of infection
6. Psychological complication due to foul smell, patient may face social problem and undergo depression.
7. Meningitis in cases of maggots (myeisis).
8. Perforation of nasal septum.

Q.9 What investigations are needed in atrophic rhinitis?

Ans. 1. Blood—for HB to detect anemia
2. VDRL—to rule out syphilis
3. X-ray chest PA view for any evidence of tuberculosis
4. X-ray PNS Water's view will show:
    - Roomy nasal chamber.
    - Atrophy of the turbinates and indistinct bony landmarks
    - Sinuses are usually small and underdeveloped with thick wall
    - Hazyness of antrum may be due to secondary sinusitis or due to thick walls of the sinuses
    - Nasal smear for leprosy and AFB
    - Biopsy usually not required, can be done if diagnosis is suspicious.
    - Antral levage: Antrum puncture in atrophic rhinites is difficult to perform because: (a) Atrum is sclerossed, so bone is hard, (b) Landmarks are lost due to crusting, (c) Atrophy of inferior turbinate so support to the canula is lost. Washing of antrum may be normal and sometimes purulent due to secondary infection.

Q.10 What are differential diagnosis of atrophic rhinitis?

Ans. Many conditions are to be differentiated including:
1. Leprosy: Lesion usually involves the cartilaginous part of septum.
2. Syphilis: Lesion usually involves the bony part of septum.
3. Rhinites sicca: Crusting only in the anterior part of the nose, no foul smelling.

4. Scleroma: Early stage, atrophic stage or may mimic the atrophic rhinitis but mucosa is pink, lesion is usually at mucocutaneous function of nasal vestibule, ala nasi is stiff and hard, nose is not roomy.
5. Rhinolith or foreign body: Hard or grity sensation to feel on probing and is unilateral.
6. Sinusitis: Crusting is absent.
7. Midline lethal granuloma.
8. Sarcoidosis.
9. Fungal granuloma.

Q.11 What is the treatment of atrophic rhinitis?

Ans. Treatment consists of:
   a. Local.
   b. Systematic.
   c. Surgical.

Q.12 What is the aim of treatment?

Ans. The aim of treatment is:
   1. Reducing crust.
   2. Reducing foul smelling.
   3. Reducing dryness and to keep the nasal cavity clean and moist.

Q.13 What is local and systematic treatment?

Ans. 1. Nasal alkaline douche: To remove the crust from the nose, to reduce the foul smell and to control the epistaxsis. Syringing of nasal cavity with warm alkaline solution by plastic syringe or by Hagginson syringe. The alkaline douche solution contains sodium chloride (for isotonic), sodium bicarbonate (for loosening the crust), and sodium bicarbonate (borax) (as an antiseptic).
   2. Nasal drops
      – 25% glucose in glycerin: Glycerin prevents drying of mucosa and glucose gets fermented into lactic acid, which prevents growth of proteolytic organisms.
      – Chloramphenicol or streptomycin nasal drops
      – Oestradiol in oil as a spray or drop
      – Mandl's paint
      – Placenta extract as a local infiltration.
   3. Systematic treatment consists of:
      – Antibiotics to control the infection.
      – Nutrition: Vitamin A and D, iron and zinc can be supplemented
      – Vasodilators for increasing the blood supply to the nose
      – Potassium iodide (orally) promotes and liquifies nasal secretion
      – Autogenious vaccine.

Q.14 What are the various surgical treatments?

Ans. 1. Autonomic surgery
   2. Repeated stellate ganglion block
   3. Cervical sympathectomy (Sharma and Sardana) to improve the blood supply of the nose

4. Submucosal grafts of:
    - Acrylic
    - Teflon
    - Dermofat from thigh
    - Cartilage
    - Bone
    - Placental bead.
5. Submucosal injection of:
    - Liquid paraffin
    - Teflon paste
    - Placenta extract
6. Witmack's operation: Transfer of stensen duct to the maxillary sinus for increasing the moisture in the nose.
7. Young's operation: Completely close nostrils, by in folding and suturing of nasal vestibule skin for about one year. It gives prolonged rest to nose and drying of nose by air current is prevented
    Disadvantages are: Patient has to breathe through the mouth and tends to snoring.
    1. Gadre's modification of Young's operation. The nostrils are completely blocked anteriorly by raising mucosal flaps and suturing them.
    2. Partial closure of nostril (Loli and Loli), 3 mm opening is left.
    3. Vestibuloplasty: (Ghosh operation) lateral folding of nasal vestibule skin like diaphragm.
    4. Endonasal microplasty.
    5. Submucosal implantation of autogeneous medullary bone graft (Chatterji) in the floor of the nose by sublabial approach
    6. Transplantation of antrum mucosa graft into the nose (Radhow sarm operation)
    7. Lantenslager's operation: Medialization of lateral wall of the nose.

Q.15 What is effect of Young's operation in atrophic rhinitis?
Ans. 1. Stratified squamous epithelium returns back to columnar ciliated.
2. Fibrosis and infiltration of lamina propria with mast cells diminish.
3. Goblet cells and mucous secreting glands increase in number and become more active.

Q.16 What are grades of atrophic rhinitis?
Ans. 1. Grade I: Atrophic change confined only to mucosa.
2. Grade II: Grade I+ partial atrophy of the turbinate bones causing roomy nose.
3. Grade III: Grade II+ almost complete atrophy of the nasal turbinates and bone with sclerotic change.

CASE: An 8-year-old child presents with increasing swelling at the frontonasal region since birth. It increases on coughing, straining and on bending forward. Swelling was nontender, firm in consistency with well-defined margins. Widening of intercanthal distance was obvious. There were multiple protuberance nodules on the swelling (Fig. 1).

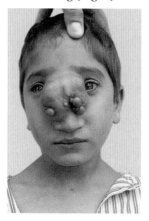

Fig. 1: Frontonasal encephalocele

Provisional Diagnosis: Frontonasal Encephalocele

Q.1 What is encephalocele?
Ans. 1. It is a congenital deformity in which intracranial contents herniated through a defect in the skull. They occur usually in the midsagittal plane from frontonasal to occipital but rarely can occur at parietal region.
   2. They are found commonly at the site of fontanelles but can appear from the defect in the cribriform plate.

Q.2 What is its classification according to their sites?
Ans. They can occur:
   1. Occipital—at or posterior to lambdoid suture.
   2. Parietal—between lambdoid coronal sutures.

3. Anterior (anterior to coronal suture):
   a. Frontonasal—(1) External; (2) Internal
   b. Frontoethmoidal
   c. Fronto-orbital
   d. Craniofacial.

Q.3 How is formed?

Ans. A defect may remain in the suture of skull bone through which meninges with some neural tissues may herniated, thus resulting in meningoencephalocele.

Q.4 What are the features of external nasal encephalocele?

Ans. 1. Present with an external swelling on the nose.
2. It is soft to firm and varies in size.
3. It may be brilliantly translucent.
4. It is usually presents at the time of birth (congenital) and increase in size as child grows.
5. Skin during the swelling is normal.
6. Pulsation may be present.
7. Swelling increases in size on coughing, crying and on straining (Furstenberg test).

Q.5 What are features of internal nasal encephalocele?

Ans. Anterior rhinoscopic examination reveals a soft, cystic, bluish, compressible translucent mass with postive Frustemberg test.

Q.6 What are investigations required?

Ans. 1. CT scan with contrast
2. MRI (skull) with contrast
3. Nasal endoscopy
4. Biopsy—should never be attempted.

Q.7 What is the finding in CT scan?

Ans. CT scan shows area of bony dehiscence with intracranial tissue in continuation through defect.

Q.8 What is the differential diagnosis?

Ans. 1. Dermoid cyst.
2. Glioma.
3. Lipoma.
4. Hemangioma.

Q.9 What is treatment of frontonasal encephalocele?

Ans. 1. Endoscopic transnasal excision (Less morbidity):
   - Closure of defect is done after removal of brain tissue if it s not reducible
   - Bone or cartilage graft is used supported with temporal fascia and fat to seal the defect
2. External approach in case frontoethmoidal meningoencephalocele
3. Craniotomy: In case of extensive cranial defect.

Rhinoscleroma

CASE: A patient presents with history of bilateral nasal obstruction with discharge of crusts. On anterior rhinoscopy granulomatous bluish red rubbery nodules are seen in the both nasal fossae. Ala nasi is stiff on palpations. The lesion commences at the mucocutaneous junction in the nasal vestibule.

Provisional Diagnosis: Rhinoscleroma

Q.1 What is rhinoscleroma?

Ans. Chronic progressive granulomatous disease of nasal mucosa extending into the nasopharynx, oropharynx and even in the larynx, trachea and bronchi. It is caused by bacillus *Klebsilla rhinoscleromatis* (Frisch bacilli). It is also called Hebra nose.

Q.2 Who described the disease?

Ans. It was described by a dermatologist of Dutch, Von Hebra. The causative organism was described by Von Frisch. Mickulicz described the characteristic foam cells in the histopathology of scleroma. Unna described the Russel bodies, seen in histological features. Professor I Fridlmann (1966) described the complete histopathogenesis of the disease in detail.

Q.3 What are histopathological features of scleroma?

Ans. Lesion consists of plasma cells, lymphocytes and eosinophils. Mikulicz cells or foam cells (in form of signet rings appearance) having vacuolated cytoplasm (with intracellular Frisch bacilli in pairs) and Russel bodies (mononuclear cell with large nucleus and scanty cytoplasm) are characteristic features. Large number of Frisch organisms are present. plasma cells get transformed into Russel's bodies.

Q.4 What are features of Frisch's bacilli?

Ans. 1. High content of mucopoly sachharides around the wall of the bacilli, protect the organism against antibiotic and antibodies.
2. Fricsh bacilli are intracellular and found in pairs.
3. Rod shaped, capsulated and nonmotile.
4. Acid-fast bacilli.

Q.5 What are etiological factors?

Ans. It mostly occurs in poor and low socioeconomic people, most commonly seen in Europe, Pakistan, Indonesia and South America.

In India, it is common in north than the south and usually seen in MP, Mumbai, Delhi, UP and Punjab.

Q.6 What are clinical features?

Ans. The disease process occurs clinically in stage from:

1. Atrophic stage: Initially there is congestion and infiltration with symptoms and sign of nasal catarrh. Subsequently changes occur in the mucosa resembling atrophic rhinitis but nose is not roomy and no anosmia. Nasal vestibule is some what stuffy. Crusting and fetor are present.

2. Nodular stage (proliferative): Bluish-red nodules appear at muco-cutaneous junction, which are rubbery in consistency. Later on these nodules become pale and hard. A cartilaginous feel of the nose is typically woody.

3. Stenotic stage (cicatrization or fibrotic stage): There is fibrosis, adhesion formation, gradually nasal cavity becomes narrow, stenosed with distortion of anatomy.

Q.7 What are peculiarities of rhinoscleromatic lesions?

Ans. 1. Rhinoscleromatic bacilli has affinity for junctional activity, so the lesion starts at the junction of change of one type of epithelium lining into another type, e.g. in nose: at nasal vestibule where squamous epithelium change into columnar ciliated epithelium.

2. In nasopharynx: Again there is change.

3. In larynx: It start at subglottic region where the squamous epithelium change into the columnar type.

4. Positive uvula sign is seen in stenosis of nasopharynx in rhinoscleroma.

Q.8 How is diagnosis confirmed?

Ans. 1. By biopsy and histological features.

2. Culture of the bacilli from biopsy material.

3. Antibodies determination.

Q.9 What are other sites where it can occur rarely?

Ans. It may involve or occur rarely in lacrimal sac, middle ear, lower part of esophagus, skin and even in the lymph node.

Q.10 What are differential diagnosis with atrophic stage of scleroma?

Ans. 1. Atrophic rhinitis: Nose is roomy, mucosa is pale, anosmia present, ala nasi is not stiff and hard. Turbinates also get atrophic and unreversible

2. Syphilis: Gumma formation, periosteum and bone are involved, nasal septal perforation.

3. Tuberculosis: Perforation of cartilaginous part of nasal septum, pain is present.

    4. Lupus vulgaris: Starts at skin and involves the mucosa, apple jelly nodules are characteristic, present over vestibule and ala of the nose.
    5. Leprosy: There is bulbous thicking of nasal vestibule, extensive crusting with foetid purulent nasal discharge.

Q.11 What is treatment of rhinoscleroma?

Ans. A long-term treatment with antibiotics (3 months) are required because:
    1. Frisch bacilli have thick mucopoly saccharide wall.
    2. Intracellular situation of bacilli.
    3. Fibrosis around the lesion does not allow blood and drug to reach to the lesion.
    4. Common antibiotics are ciprofloxacin, doxycyclin, terramycin, chloramphenicol, minicyclin, etc.
    5. Surgery may be needed to excise the stenotic and obliterating lesion.

Q.12 Why scleroma not commonly involves lymph node?

Ans. In scleroma of nose, pharynx and larynx, the lymphadenitis is rare because:
    1. Organisms are intracellular.
    2. Fibrosis and scarring may block the lymphatics.

Q.13 What are features by which atrophic stage of rhinoscleroma can be differentiated by primary atrophic rhinites?

Ans. In atrophic stage of scleroma:
    1. The nasal cavity is not roomy.
    2. Stiffness of the ala nasal is present.
    3. Fetor is not marked.

CASE

58

Rhinosporidiosis

CASE: A patient presents with history of progressive nasal obstruction and nasal discharge of 6 months duration. He also has episodes of bleeding from the same nose. Anterior rhinoscopy reveals a soft non-tender, irregular reddish mass resembling a strawberry with multiple nodules on its surface (Fig. 1).

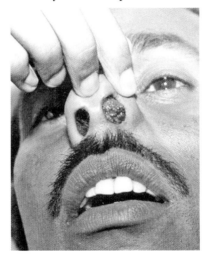

Fig. 1: Rhinosporidiosis in left nasal fossa

Provisional Diagnosis: Rhinosporidiosis

Q.1 What is rhinosporidiosis?
Ans. It is a noncontagious, chronic condition caused by *Rhinosporidiosis seeberi* or *R. kinealyi* a spore-bearing fungus, which affect mainly the nose.

Q.2 What is the mode of infection?
Ans. 1. Infection is from the dust and dung of infected horse and cattle which caries spores of the fungus.
2. By contact with contaminated water while bathing.

Q.3 In which part it is common?

Ans. It is common in South India, Ceylon, Africa, America and Italy.

In India, it is common in Kerala, Tamil Nadu, Andhra Pradesh, Odisha (Cuttack and Ganjam) and MP (Raipur and Durg district). In Rajasthan, it is common in Udaipur region.

Q.4 What is the historical aspect of rhinosporidiosis?

Ans. Malbran saw the first case affecting the nose of an Italian agriculture worker during the year 1892. Subsequently, Major O'Kinaly reported a case from India (Calcutta) in a young worker in raw hides and skins in 1897. Later Seeber (1900) described this disease by way of dissertations, in Spanish language to the faculty of medicine, University of Buenos Aires, Argentina.

Q.5 What is the gross pathology?

Ans. Polypoidal masses are formed in the nose, which are very vascular. Grossly they are reddish, friable, pedunculated or sessile. When sessile the mass appears as multiple nodules or may assume a leaf shape with rounded or dentate sporangia: are scattered in the vascular masses. They are chitinous cysts containing spores.

Q.6 What are commons sites of origin?

Ans. It arises primarily in the vestibule and usually from the nasal septum (Little' area) and it may spread backwards into the nasopharynx and even hang into the oropharynx. Other common sites are skin, conjunction the eyelid.

Q.7 What are common symptoms?

Ans. 1. Nasal obstruction: Common.
2. Epistaxis: Frequent.
3. Rhinorrhea: May be present.
4. Protrusion of mass through nares.

Q.8 What are clinical features?

Ans. 1. The nose contains a gray red colored mulberry-like polypoidal mass which is mobile, soft, nontender, attached to nasal septum or turbinate, with bleeding tendency on probing and friable.
2. Sporangia are seen as minute grayish spots particularly on the under surface of the mass.

Q.9 How does it spread?

Ans. Along with nasal involvement: The eyes, pharynx, trachea, and genitals may be occasionally affected.

Q.10 What is the histological picture of rhinosporidiosis?

Ans. It is a vascular myxomatous structure. There are round or oval cells containing the sporangia in the stoma. The epithelium covering the lesion shows capillary process. The subepithelium tissues is very vascular with young newly developed capillary with infiltration of polymorphs, lymphocytes, plasma cells and red cells.

Fully developed sporangia are found on the external surface while the developing one are deep inside. Giant cells are rarely seen.

Q.11 How will you confirm the clinical diagnosis?

Ans. 1. Smear: It is examined under microscope with a drop of 5% KOH, over the smear. Typically double-walled cysts of about 300 microns size, filled with innumerable spores is diagnostic.
Alcian blue stains both cyst wall and the wall of the spores.
2. Biopsy: Typical features.

Q.12 What is the treatment of rhinosporidiosis?

Ans. 1. Radical surgery with surrounding healthy tissue and cauterization of the base.
2. Topical application of emetine, tolnaftate 2% solution and antimony tartrate has variable results.
3. Systematic therapy:
   a. Dapsone over a prolonged period—delay the recurrence.
   b. Amphotericin B.
4. Local infection of depo-corticosteroids—into the polypoidal masses.
5. Cryosurgery.
6. Laser: May be used with minimal bleeding.
7. Endoscopic surgery: Help to identify the pedicle and thus reduce the chances of recurrence after excision.

Q.13 Why cavity is done after removal of rhinosporidiosis?

Ans. 1. To minimize the recurrence by destroying the spores.
2. To stop hemorrhage.

Q.14 Why is piecemeal tissue removal avoided in rhinosporidiosis?

Ans. To prevent hematogenous spread as all patients with generalized disease has a history of previous surgery.

Q.15 What is differential diagnosis of strawberry type of nasal mass?

Ans. These can be:
1. Rhinoscleroma.
2. Inverted papilloma.
3. Adenocystic carcinoma.
4. Multiple nasal polyps.

CASE

59   Juvenile Nasopharyngeal Angiofibroma

CASE : A male child of 10 years presents with history of nasal obstruction and recurrent episode of epistaxis. On examination, there is bulging of the soft palate. Postnasal mirror examination reveals fleshy mass, angry red in color in the nasopharynx, over which blood vessels traveling are also seen (Fig. 1).

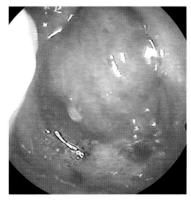

Fig. 1: Endoscopic view of nasopharyngeal angiofibroma

Provisional Diagnosis: Juvenile Nasopharyngeal Angiofibroma

Q.1 What is the diagnosis?
Ans. Provisional diagnosis: Juvenile nasopharyngeal angiofibroma (JNA).

Q.2 What is a juvenile nasopharyngeal angiofibroma?
Ans. Juvenile nasopharyngeal angiofibroma is a benign, highly vascular tumor with aggressive nature with a tendency to spread in the adjoining cavities and spaces. Clinically, it presents with triad of nasal obstruction, recurrent epistaxsis and a nasopharyngeal mass in young adolescent males.

Q.3 What are etiological factors?
Ans. 1. JNA is less than 0.05% of head and neck tumors.
      2. Geographical: More common in South East Asia and Middle East and also common in India.

3. Sex: Almost exclusively in males.
4. Age: Common in puberty age, young age between 10–20 years (mean age 14 years).
5. Endocrines: Common in puberty age, regressive with advancing age, therapeutic effects of sex hormones.
6. Immune response.
7. Metabolic disorder: Common in growth period.
8. Overgrowth of fetal eractile tissue (hamartomatous origin).

Q.4 What is its pathogenesis?

Ans. Several tissues have been claimed for its origin.

1. Ringert's theory: Periostium of nasopharyngeal—vault inequality growth of bones of skull base resulted from hypertrophy of underlying periostium in response to hormonal influence.
2. Benschanct Ewing: Arises from embryonic fibrocartilagious disc between the basiocciput and basisphenoid.
3. Som and Neffson: Suggestive hypertrophy of periosteum under hormonal influence.
4. Bunner: Origin from conjoined pharyngobasilar and buccopharyngeal fascia.
5. Osborn: Considered it to be hamartoma of residual of fetal eractile tissue.
6. Girgis and Fahmy: Arises from the paraganglionic cells around the terminal part of maxillary artery (fore-runners of angiomata), i.e. one short of parangioma or chemodectoma (presence of cells of Zella Ballan).
7. Angiomata arising from vestiges of the atrophied stapedial artery.

Q.5 What are the sites of origin of nasopharyngeal fibroma?

Ans. It arises from:

1. Medial wall and margins of sphenopalatine foramen.
2. Vault of nasopharynx.
3. Choana.
4. Pterygoid apophysis.
5. Sphenoid.

Q.6 What is the gross pathology?

Ans. The mass is firm, spongy, lobulated swelling, nodularity increases with age. Color varies from pink to white. Cut section shows reticulated whorled or spongy appearance and no true capsule but well-defined edge.

Q.7 What is the histological picture of nasopharyngeal fibroma?

Ans. It has three components :

1. Vascular: This contains two types of vessels normal blood vessel and fetal type of blood vessel. Blood vessels of embryonic type (deficit of middle muscular layer in the wall, so lack of contractile) are large, thin sinosoidal vessels of varying size lined by flattened epithelium. Later on there may be intravascular thrombosis in some vessels. Bleeding commonly occurs because the vessels do not contract.

2. Stroma: Coarse parallel wavy or interlocking of collagen in which stromal cells are seen to radiate outward from the vessels.
3. Undifferentiated epithelial cells "Zellaballan" at the growing edge of the tumor.

Q.8 What are the types of blood vessels which supply the tumor?

Ans. The feeding vessels of angiofibroma are:
1. Internal maxillary artery, is enlarged and is main feeding vessel.
2. Ascending pharyngeal artery.
3. Vidian artery.
4. Unnamed branches of internal carotid artery.
5. Branches of vertebral artery, rarely.

Q.9 How is nasopharyngeal angiofibroma classified according to location and extension?

Ans. Classification (Sission et al. 1981).
1. Stage I: Tumor limited to nasopharyngeal vault
2. Stage II:
   a. Minimal lateral extension through sphenopalatine foramen into pterygopalatine fossa.
   b. Extension to pterygopalatine wall of the antrum or superior extension eroding bone of orbit.
   c. Through pterygomaxillary fossa to extension into cheek or temporal fossa.
3. State III: Intracranial extension (only in 20–25%).

Stage II and III are difficult to manage. Recurrence is common in stage III.

Q.10 What are clinical features of nasopharyngeal fibroma?

Ans. 1. Epistaxis: Recurrent and severe (in 70–90%).
2. Nasal obstruction: Progessive, unilateral initially but later on bilaterally (80–90%).
3. Nasal discharge: Mucopurulent.
4. Conductive deafness (3–13%) due to Eustachian tube obstruction.
5. Hyposmia or anosmia.
6. Nasal speech (rhinolalia clausa): Due to nasal obstruction.
7. Facial deformity (in 13–20%): In late stage.
8. Headache: Due to blocked sinuses.
9. Proptosis (8–13%): In late state.
10. Other symptoms: Trismus, defective vision, purulent secretion with DNS toward healthy side.

Q.11 What are various findings in nasopharyngeal fibroma?

Ans. 1. Anterior rhinoscopy: If nasal extension a fleshy mass, angry red in color with blood vessels overlying the surface. It is soft-to-firm in consistency.
2. Posterior rhinoscopy: A fleshy mass, angry red to pink in color seems to arising from the roof of the nasopharynx.

3. Oral cavity examination: Bulging of soft palate (3–10%) in case of large tumor, thickening of the area between side of maxilla and ascending ramous of the mandible and trismus.
4. External examination of the nose and face proptosis (3–13%), broadening of nasal bridge (frog-face deformity), cheek swelling, (buccal and temporal extension), impaired vision, bulging of the parotid region.

Q.12 How does nasopharyngeal angiofibroma extend and spread?

Ans. Nasopharyngeal angiofibroma arises from the medial surface of sphenopalatine foramen and then it spreads in all directions.

1. Lateral extension: By various routes nasopharynx to through spenopalatine foramen:
   a. To pterygopalatine fossa to maxillary antrum.
   b. Through infraorbital fissure to orbit.
   c. Through pterygomaxillary fissure to cheek and temporal region.
   d. Fascia basilis and sinus of Morgagni to infratemporal fossa.
2. Forward extension: Various routes:
   a. Nasopharynx: To through choana to nasal cavity to maxillary antrum to orbit.
   b. Nasal cavity to ethmoidal sinus breaking lamina papyracca to orbit.
3. Backwards-upward extension route:
   a. Nasopharynx: To sphenoid sinus to pituitaty fossa.
   b. Nasopharynx: Eroding greater wing of sphenoid into middle cranial fossa.
   c. Nasopharynx: Through cribriform plate to anterior cranial fossa.
   d. Nasopharynx: foramen lacerun to middle cranial fossa.

Q.13 What are the criteria's and investigations for diagnosis of nasopharyngeal fibroma?

Ans. 1. Clinical: Always be diagnosed clinically.
2. Biopsy should be avoided and is indicated only when there are signs of neurological involvement.
3. Fundus: To exclude intracranial extension
4. Radiological:
   i. X-ray: (a) Lateral view of the nasopharyx—soft tissue shadow arising from roof; (b) X-ray PNS water's view—soft tissue shadow with evidence of bone absorption; (c) X-ray lateral view of PNS. Anterior bowing of the posterior wall of the antrum (antral sign); (d) X-ray base of skull (axial or Hurst view).
   ii. CT scan: Contrast enhanced CT scan is the investigation of choice.
   iii. MRI.
   iv. Carotid angiography.

Q.14 What are the radiological findings in nasopharyngcal fibroma?

Ans. Findings are:
1. Soft tissue mass in nasopharynx (Fig. 2).

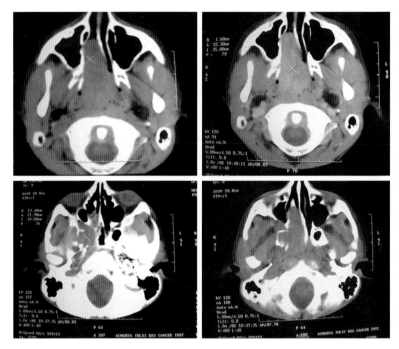

Fig. 2: CT scan: Showing soft tissue mass involving right posterior nasal cavity extending into the nasopharynx with widening of pterygopalatine fossa with erosion of pterygoid lamina with extension into the sphenoid cavity

2. Antral sign, anterior bowing of the posterior wall of the maxilla Hollman' Miller sign is pathognomic.
3. Erosion of base of medial pterygoid (Fig. 2) with enlargement of sphenopalatine foramen (Leyod and Phelps).
4. Postetior bowing pterygoid plate is classical sign.
5. Widening of pterygoid fissure or sphenopalatine foramen.
6. Widening of superior orbital fissure with proptosis.
7. Opacity of invasion, erosion of sinuses with displacement of nasal septum to opposite side.
8. Erosion of sphenoid sinuses and erosion of medial wall of antrum.
9. Erosion of hard palate.
10. Erosion of medial pterygoid plate.

Q.15 What are the indications of carotid angiography in nasopharyngeal fibroma?

Ans. 1. To detect the volume and extension of the lesion.
2. To detect the feeding vessel of tumor.
3. To detect the vascularity pattern.
4. Indicated prior to embolization procedure.

Q.16 What is differential diagnosis of nasopharyngeal fibroma?

Ans. 1. Hypertrophic adenoid.
2. Antrochoanal polyp.
3. Malignant tumor.

4. Choanal polyp.
5. Basisphenoid cordoma.
6. Craniopharyngioma.
7. Glioma.
8. Menigoencephalocele.
9. Dermoid cyst.
10. Mucous cyst.
11. Thornwaldt bursitis.
12. Hemangioma.
13. Teratoma.
14. Inverted papilloma.

Q.17 What are various modalities of treatment of nasopharyngeal fibroma?
Ans. 1. Surgery.
2. Radiotherapy.
3. Hormonal therapy.

Q.18 What are the indications of radiotherapy in nasopharyngeal fibroma?
Ans. Radiotherapy cobalt 60 can be given in:
1. Curative dose (4000–6000 reds): In inoperable cases, rapidly growing with intracranial extension or recurrent tumor.
2. Sclerosing dose (2000–4000 reds): Preoperative in advanced cases to increase collagen formation and decrease vascularity.
   Radiotherapy in young age is hazardous because of chances of development of malignancy and osteomyelitis, later on.

Q.19 What are the indications of hormone in nasopharyngeal fibroma and its disadvantage or side-effects?
Ans. Indications:
1. To decrease the vascularity and size of the tumor (pre-operatively) in extensive tumor.
2. Minor recurrence.
Various hormoncs are used for about 1 month period
1. Estrorgen: 5 mg TDS (side-effect are gynecomastia and generalized pruritis).
2. Testosterone.
3. Gonadotropins.

Q.20 What are various modalities of surgery in nasopharyngeal angiofibroma?
Ans. 1. Cryosurgery: By nitrogen gas.
2. Laser beam surgery: Stage I
3. Endoscopic surgery: Stage I and II b.
4. Classical surgery.
5. Electrocoagulative.

Q.21 What are various surgical approaches for extraction of nasopharyngeal fibroma?

Ans. 1. Transpalatine (Wilson's): If lesion confined to nasopharyngeal region.
   2. Lateral rhinotomy (Moore's): If main mass in nasal cavity.
   3. Runge Denker approach.
   4. Transzygomatic for temporal extension.
   5. Transmandible.
   6. Transmaxillary: In maxillary extension lesion.
   7. Broca's approach.
   8. Sublabial mid gloves (Shaheen approach).
   9. Mid-maxillary with Weber Ferguson.
   10. Neurocraniotomy: For intracranial excision.

Q.22 What are various measures to reduce the bleeding in nasopharyngeal fibroma?

Ans. Preoperative measures:
   1. Radiotherapy: Sclerosing dose.
   2. Hormone therapy.
   3. Microembolization (gel foam paste or micropieces injected that block the veins).
   4. Antidromic blood transfusion: Blood transfusion against the arterial flow (Phenomenon of pastilles).
   5. Blood transfusion.
   6. Hypotensive anesthesia: (a) Nitroproside; (b) Trimetaphen. BP is lowered up to 60 mm mercury systolic for about 15–20 minutes during operation.
   7. External carotid artery ligation just before operation.
   Postsurgery measures:
   1. Muscle graft in fossa (vastuslateralis piece) or bone wax.
   2. Posterior nasal pack.
   3. Anterior nasal pack.
   4. Blood transfusion.

Q.23 What are complications of surgery?

Ans. 1. Palatal fistula (in Wilson approach).
   2. Anesthesia of cheek (infraorbital nerve section).
   3. Slight ectropion of lower lid.
   4. Nasal crusting.
   5. Nasal stenosis.

Q.24 Why does nasopharyngeal angiofibroma bleed profusely?

Ans. There is lack of contractile power in blood vessels of the tumor. These are embryonic type, i.e. deficit of tunica media (muscular layer) in the wall of vessels.

CASE

60 Nasopharyngeal Carcinoma

CASE: A 12-year-old boy presented with history of nasal obstruction and recurrent episodes of epistaxis and swelling on the left side of neck. Examination revealed left side nasal air way obstruction and endoscopy revealed a mass in the nasopharynx. Neck examination revealed left cervical lymphadenopathy which is somewhat hard and non-tender.

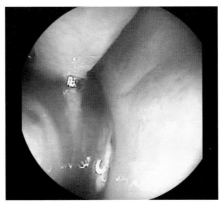

Fig.1: Endoscopic view of growth

Provisional Diagnosis: Nasopharyngeal Carcinoma

Q.1 What is provisional diagnosis?
Ans. Nasopharyngeal carcinoma.

Q.2 What are points in favor of diagnosis?
Ans. Carcinoma nasopharynx has bimodal presentation, i.e. between 10–20 years and later at about 50–65 years of age.
   History of progressive obstruction and recurrent episode of bleeding and painless cervical lymphadenopathy (metastatic). A reddish mass in nasopharynx on postmirror examination and also on rigid endoscopy.

Q.3 What are the etiological factors for carcinoma nasopharynx?
Ans. It is caused by a combination of factors just like for germination, growth and development of plants, three things are required, i.e. soil, seed and

environment (like water, fertilizer, climate, etc). Similarly for development of carcinoma, the soil is tissue of the body, i.e. genetic peculiarity, seed, i.e. causative organism, here it is thought to be Epstein-Barr virus (EBV). Environmental factors are age, diet, cooking habits, occupation, nutritional deficiencies, socioeconomic status, tobacco, etc.

Q.4 What is geographical distribution of the disease?

Ans. 1. It comprises 2% of all malignant tumors of head and neck, but its incidence in China is as high as 18% of all malignant tumors.
2. It is more common in Southern China (Kwantung Province), Hong Kong, Taiwan, South-East Asian races (Malay, Kadazan, Iban), Bidayuh, Indonesians and Thias and also Eskimos, North Africa and Tunisia.
3. The incidence is high in these groups even after migration to other countries where there is low incidence, however 2nd and 3rd generation born in USA, shows declined incidence. Its incidence is lower among mongoloid race such as Northern Chinese, Koreans and Japanese.

Q.5 What are various environmental factors for carcinoma of the nasopharynx?

Ans. These are:
1. Age: Among Chinese it is common between 15–20 years of age and then between 35–64 years and subsequently incidence sharply declines. Among low risk populations it has bimodal presentation, i.e. between 10–20 years and later on between 55–65 years of age.
2. Sex: It is more common among males with ratio of 3:1.
3. Tabacco smoking.
4. Chinese herbal medicine.
5. Diet: Salted fish, persevered vegetables, spicy meat, fermented food.
6. Occupation: Industrial fumes, chemical, formaldehyde, wood dust, exposure to nickel, chromium and radioactive metals.
7. Cooking habits: House hold smoke and fumes.
8. Religious practices: In-sense and joss stick smoke.
9. Socioeconomic status: Nutritional deficiencies like vitamin A and C.

Q.6 What is Epstein-Barr virus?

Ans. It is most common worldwide and easily spreading virus. Ninety-five percent of all people in United States are exposed to this virus by the time of the age between 30–40 years. Very rarely does EB virus lead to cancer, which suggests a variety of influencing factors like genetic susceptibility and other environmental factors. EBV DNA is present in 96% of patients with nonkeratinizing nasopharyngeal carcinoma in the blood plasma. Moderate to well-differentiated carcinoma are devoid of EB virus antigen.

Q.7 What is histological classification of nasopharyngeal carcinoma?

Ans. WHO classified it into:
1. WHO Type-1: Well-differentiated squamous cell carcinoma (Keratinizing type).

2. WHO Type -2: Nonkeratinizing type resembling transitional cell type.
3. WHO Type-3: Undifferentiated carcinoma:
   a. Lymphoepithelioma.
   b. Anaplastic carcinoma.

The new WHO classification in relation to EB virus association.

1. Type-1: Keratinizing squamous cell carcinoma.
2. Type-2: Nonkeratinizing carcinoma
   a. Differentiated.
   b. Undifferentiated.

Q.8 How does the tumor grossely presents?

Ans. Usually the tumor presents in several forms.
1. Proliferative growth causing nasal obstruction.
2. Ulcerative causing epistaxis.
3. Mixed.
4. Infiltrative which causes cranial nerve involvement.

Q.9 What are various symptoms of the carcinoma of nasopharynx?

Ans. The symptoms depend on type and site of involvement and extension of the growth.
1. Cervical: Lump in the neck (60–80%) is most common presenting symptoms.
2. Nasal symptoms: Nasal obstruction, epistaxis and other nasorespiration in about 40%.
3. Otological symptoms: Present in about 30% which is due to Eustachian tube obstruction. These are blocked ear, hearing loss, painful ear, tinnitus.
4. Neurological symptoms: In about 20% includes headache, cranial nerve palsy and Horner's syndrome.
5. Ophthalmic symptoms like epiphora, diplopia.
6. Miscellaneous: Like weightloss, anorexia, trismus, weakness.
7. Trotter's triad: Classical.

Q.10 What is trotter's triad?

Ans. Triad of symptoms in patients with carcinoma nasopharynx constitutes:
1. Conductive deafness due to middle ear effusion (tube obstruction).
2. Facial pain due to trigeminal nerve involvement at foramen ovale.
3. Local invasion of the palate may cause immobility (tight palate) or paralysis of soft palate may be due to involvement of cranial accessory nerve in pharyngeal plexus through vagus.

Q.11 What are common sites of origin of nasopharyngeal carcinoma?

Ans. Common sites are the lateral wall or super lateral wall of the nasopharynx around fossa of Rosenmüller.

Q.12 What is fossa of Rosenmüller?

Ans. It is also known as posterior lateral recess. It is located superior and posterior to the torus tuberi (posterior projection of cartilaginous portion of Eustachian tube) and is formed by mucosal reflection over the longus colli muscle.

Q.13 How does the tumor spread?

Ans. Nasopharyngeal carcinoma spread by direct, lymphatic and hematogenous routes.

Q.14 How does it spread by direct mode?

Ans. It can spread into all directions.

1. Anteriorly to nasal cavity, paranasal sinuses and orbit and also pterygopalatine and infratemporal fossa through sphenopalatine foramen.
2. Posteriorly to retropharyngeal space and node of Rouviere, destroys lateral mass of atlas.
3. Laterally to parapharyngeal space through sinus of Morgagni and can involve both pre- and post-styloid compartment. In post-styloid compartment it causes vascular compression of carotid sheath, invasion of last four cranial nerves (especially IX, X are most commonly involved) and cervical sympathetic nerves.

Inferiorly: It spreads into oral cavity and retrotonsillar regions.

Superiorly: It extends into the intracranial cavity by eroding the base of skull or through foramen, especially foramen of lacerum, which lies close to the fossa of Rosenmüller so it can easily spread into the cranial cavity (Linconi highway). The over route of spread is petrosphenoid route in which growth invades the petrosa or occipit or surrounding sphenoid and reaches early to involve cavernous sinus and its contents.

Advanced growth may extend anteriorly along middle cranial fossa involving the optic nerve and orbit.

Posterior fossa involvement is rare. The tumor may also destroy directly basi sphenoid, basi occiput and petrous temporal bone and sella turcica to optic chiasma and then to extend to the orbit through the superior orbital fissure to cause proptosis.

Q.15 How does the lymphatic spread occur in nasopharyngeal carcinoma?

Ans. Lymphatic pathway can be divided into median and lateral groups.

1. The median group: Drains the roof and the posterior wall of nasopharynx into the retropharyngeal node, which may be by passed so the first noticeable lymph node metastasis is the upper deep cervical group of lymph nodes.
2. The lateral group: Drains the lateral nasopharynx including the fossa of Rosenmüller. The lymphatics drain into the upper internal jugular chain or into lateral retropharyngeal node (Node of Rouviere). It usually lies below the base of skull near the level of atlas and may overlay the internal carotid artery. The upper cervical lymph node receive lymph from the node of Rouviere. Then from upper cervical lymph node the metastasis occurs into the lower deep cervical groups. The last four cranial nerve may be involved at jugular foramen.

Q.16 What is jugular foramen syndrome?

Ans. The last four cranial nerves may be involved in malignancy of the nasopharynx due to:

1. Compression by the node metastasis close to jugular foramen (node of Krause).
2. From metastasis in upper deep cervical lymph node.
3. From direct involvement of deep pharyngeal recess at base of skull.

The IX, X and XI are involved at jugular foramen while the XII nerve may be involved by growth extending to hypoglossal canal.

Q.17 Which metastatic lymph nodes are commonly palpable in nasopharyngeal carcinoma?
Ans. Retropharyngeal group (Rouviere): Not palpable.

Commonest palpable nodes are: Jugulodiagastric, preaccessory, posterior triangle, HO's triangle, supraclavicular (L2/L3/L5 level). Contralateral lymph node: May be the site of metastasis as nasopharynx is midline structure.

Q.18 How does nasopharyngeal carcinoma spread by hematogenous route?
Ans. The incidence rate is about 30%: Distant metastasis occurs commonly to bone like thoracolumbar spine (50%), lung and liver.

Q.19 How the facial nerve is involved in nasopharyngeal carcinoma?
Ans. It can be involved by several routes: By extension of growth through Eustachian tube, by direct erosion of petrous temporal bone during intracranial invasion, by metastasis in temporal bone or by metastasis in parotid groups of lymph node.

Q.20 What is TNM classification for nasopharyngeal carcinoma?
Ans. Primary tumor
1. T1—Tumor confined to nasopharynx.
2. T2a—Tumor extends to oropharynx/nasal cavity without parapharyngeal spread.
3. T2b—Tumor with parapharyngeal extension.
4. T3—Tumor involves bony structures and/or paranasal sinuses.
5. T4—Tumor invasion intracranial structures and/or cranial nerves, infratemporal fossa, orbit, masticator space or hypopharynx.

N: Cervical lymph node involvement
1. N0—No clinically positive node
2. N1—Single clinically positive hemolateral node 3 cm or less in diameter.
3. N2—Single clinically positive homolateral node >3 cm but <6 cm or multiple clinically positive homolateral nodes >6 cm in diameter.
4. N3—Massive homolateral node(s), bilateral nodes or contralateral node(s).

M: Distant metastasis
1. MX—Not assessed
2. M0—No (Known) distant metastasis
3. M1—Distant metastasis present.

Q.21 What are the investigations to be done?

Ans. 1. Diagnostic nasal endoscopy: To examine nasopharynx, localization and extent of growth and biopsy under vision.
2. FNAC: From metastatic lymph node.
3. CT Scan: To know extent of growth and neck node metastasis.
4. Bone scan: For metastasis.
5. USG of the abdomen: For liver metastasis.
6. MRI: Gives better soft tissue view.
7. X-ray chest PA: For lung metastasis.
8. X-ray base of skull (axial view): May occasionally be useful. Distortion in the line of Beclizzae in the base of skull view gives a rough idea about tumor spread.
9. Positron emission tomography (PET) imaging: Used to assess questionable neck nodes and evaluate for other sites of distant disease.
10. Epstein-Barr virus (EBV) titer including immunoglobulin G (IgG) and immunoglobulin A (IgA) antibodies to the viral capsid antigen, early antigen and nuclear antigen should be performed. These titer may correlate with tumor burden and decrease with treatment.

Q.22 What is the treatment of nasopharyngeal carcinoma?

Ans. Combination of radiotherapy and chemotherapy.
1. Radiotherapy: Definitive treatment. Field, from base of skull to entire neck up to clavicle is included, i.e. disease in the primary site and neck lymph adenopathy (Level 1 to 5 neck nodes are included).
2. Brachy therapy: Transnasal intracavity brachy therapy with iridium–192 is used.

Chemotherapy: Concurrent cisplatin, 5-fluorouracil is helpful in improving survival.

Q.23 What is the differential diagnosis of nasopharyngeal carcinoma?

Ans. It should be differentiated from:
1. Non-Hodgkin's lymphoma.
2. Nasopharyngeal fibroma.
3. Sarcoma.
4. Plasmacytoma.
5. Enlarged adenoid (in cases of children).
6. Intranasal glioma.
7. Chordoma.
8. Craniopharyngioma.
9. Meningoencephalocele.
10. Adenocystic carcinoma.
11. Minor salivary gland tumor.
12. Nasal polyps.
13. Pediatric rhabdomyosarcoma.

Q.24 What is prognosis of nasopharyngeal carcinoma?

Ans. Five-year survival is 45–50%. Local recurrence and distant metastasis occurs in about 90% in 2–3 years.

Dentigerous Cyst and Ameloblastoma

CASE: Slow growing, painless swelling causing expansion of the bone. Thin bone shows sign of egg-shell cracking. Tooth is missing at the site of swelling.

Provisional Diagnosis: Dentigerous Cyst (Follicular Cyst or Odontome)

Q.1 What is dentigerous cyst?

Ans. It is developmental odontogenic cyst arising from the enamel organ (epithelium) in the crown of a permanent developing tooth (after amelogenesis has been completed). The expanding cyst is formed from the follicle (consisting of an inner epithelial layer and outer connective tissue covering, so it is also called follicular cyst). The root remains unerupt and remained impacted in the cyst or its wall. It constitutes 95% of follicular cysts and 34% of odontogenic cysts.

Q.2 Which tooth is commonly affected?

Ans. The third molar in the mandible and premolar (cuspid) in the maxilla.

Q.3 How does cyst form and expand?

Ans. 1. First separation of the enamel epithelium from the surface of the crown of the unerupted tooth occurs.
2. Fluid accumulate to form cystic swelling.
3. The cyst enlarges with expansion of bone and displacement of attached tooth.
4. The cyst wall is thick, may contain patches of calcified tissue and lined fibrous tissue, stratified squamous or columnar epithelium.
5. Cyst is usually solitary and may occasionally be multilocular, and contains an unerupted tooth.

Q.4 What are radiological features?

Ans. A well-circumscribed radiolucent area is seen with clearly defined margin and unerupted tooth in the cavity. Sometime, there may be a peripheral scale of sclerosis surrounding the translucent area. At times pseudo-trabecular pattern (soap-bubble appearance) in translucent area is seen.

Q.5 What are complications of dentigerous cyst?
Ans. 1. Transformation into ameloblastoma.
2. Pain due to pressure in the root of adjacent tooth.

Q.6 What is the treatment of dentigerous cyst?
Ans. Enucleation along with the tooth of origin (Fig. 1).

Q.7 What are other odontogenic cysts?
Ans. 1. Radicular cyst (apical periodontal cyst): Results from infection of the root canal following long chronic inflammation in periapical granuloma.
2. Primordial cyst: It develops as a cystic degeneration occurring prior to maturation of enamel organ.

Q.8 What are odontogenic neoplasms?
Ans. Tumors arise from dental lamina (early ectoderm invagination into the jaws) or any of its derivatives.

Q.9 What are other cysts arising from jaw?
Ans. These are embryological fusion cyst:
1. Lateral alveolar cyst.
2. Nasopalatine cyst.
3. Median alveolar cyst.
4. Nasoalveolar cyst.
5. Median palatal cyst.

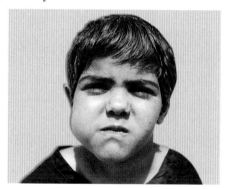

Fig. 1: Swelling of right cheek due to dentigerous cyst

Q.10 What are odontogenic tumors?
Ans. Tumors arising from the enamel or tooth forming cells (ameloblast) or from the tooth tissue. These can be classified as follows:
1. Benign tumors: Adenomatoid tumor, calcifying epithelial tumor, ameloblastic fibroma and odontoma (not invastive) do not recur following simple excision. Associated with unerupted tooth.

2. Borderline tumor: Ameloblastoma .
3. Malignant tumor: Ameloblastic carcinoma and fibrosarcoma (Fig. 2).

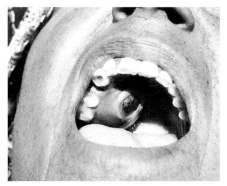

Fig. 2: Palato-alveolar swelling due to odontogenic tumor

Q.11 What is ameloblastoma?

Ans. 1. It is benign but borderline odontogenic tumor arising from the ameloblast that is from enamel organ as a result of failure of differentiation.
2. Ameloblastoma is also called adamantinoma, adamantine epithelioma, multicystic disease of jaw, and fibrocystic disease of jaw, Eve's disease.

Q.12 What are features of ameloblastoma?

Ans 1. Slow growing, locally invasive, low grade (or potentialy malignant) epithelial tumor.
2. High recurrence following inadequate removal.
3. No tendency to metastasize.
4. Arises
   a. ameloblast (primitive enamel forming cell) from the embryonic enamel organ of tooth as a result of failure of differentiation.
   b. Stratified squamous epithelium of the oral cavity or displaced dental epithelial remnants.
   c. From the dentigerous cyst (20%).
5. It is common in 4th and 5th decade and in female.
6. Painless progressive swelling prominent externally of the jaw, lobulated surface, soft fluctuant or egg-shell cracking with mal-alignment of teeth, no missing tooth.
7. No regional lymph node enlargement.
8. Radiologically: Radiolucent area separated by bony septa or trabeculae of varying size give honey-comb or soap-bubble appearance, some time moth-eaten irregularity along edge (Fig. 3).
9. It is rare tumor, accounting for only 2% of all tumors and cysts of the jaw.
10. Treatment is radical surgery because of its nature of high recurrence and potential malignant.

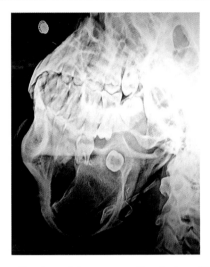

Fig. 3: Large unilocular radiolucent expending shadow of the mandible

Q.13 Which skin carcinoma resembles with ameloblastoma?

Ans. The ameloblastoma cells resemble basal cell of skin cancer 'basal cell carcinoma'. The clinical behavior of an ameloblastoma also resembles that of basal cell carcinoma, both tumors are slow growing and locally invasive and have a limited metastatic potential.

Q.14 What are histological features of ameloblastoma?

Ans. Histologically, the tumor has a characteristic pattern of follicles lined by tall columnar cells with reversed nuclear polarity. The epithelium is supported by a mature collageneous stroma.

Q.15 What are basic treatment modalities of the odontogenic cysts or tumors?

Ans. These are:
1. Simple enucleation, with or without curettage—used in more benign lesions.
2. Marginal or segmental resection of the lesion and surrounding bone—indicated in benign but more locally invasive lesions.
3. Composite resection of bones and surrounding soft tissue—used in malignant tumor.

CASE: A 45-year-old man presents with swelling on the right side of cheek region with history of progressive right side nasal obstruction and episodes of bleeding right side nose and nasal discharge for 6 months duration and swelling on the right side of face on the outer surface of cheek. Anterior rhinoscopy reveal a fleshy nontender mass arising from lateral wall of the nose. It bleeds on touch, friable and occupying the nasal fossa. Orbital surface of maxilla was not affected and found to have sharp margin, smooth surface nontender and freely mobile skin over it. Oral cavity examination revealed slight fullness in right gingivolabial sulcus. All teeth were normal, no pain, no loose teeth. No trismus, hard palate and soft palate were normal. Posterior rhinoscopy was also normal. Neurological examination was normal except slight decreased sensation on the right cheek. Cervical lymph nodes were not palpable.

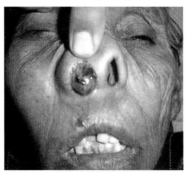

Fig. 1: Growth protruding in the right nasal cavity

Provisional Diagnosis: Sinonasal Tumors

Q.1 What is the diagnosis?

Ans. Provisional diagnosis: Tumor right maxilla.

Q.2 What are various points in favor of diagnosis?

Ans. It is tumor of the right maxilla—possibly a malignant neoplasm. Maxilla has five surfaces. All surfaces are examined:

1. Superficial or anterolateral surface: Patient has a swelling progressively increasing, nontender on the right side of cheek with no sign of inflammation (Figs 2 and 3).

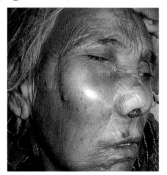

Fig. 2: Swelling of the right cheek due to cancer maxillary antrum

2. Orbital or superior surface is examined and compared with opposite side. Normally, the inferior orbital margin is sharp and smooth while in case of its involvement it becomes blunt, rough and uneven. Normally, orbital surface is nontender, skin overlying is free and there is no chemosis of conjunctiva. In case of affection, it becomes tender, skin is fixed and there may be chemosis of conjunctiva (Fig. 3).

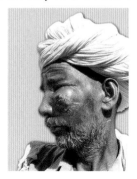

Fig. 3: Swelling lift face region due to growth of maxillary antrum

3. Nasal or medial surface is examined by anterior and posterior rhinoscopy. In this case, anterior rhinoscopy reveals a fleshy red colored mass (Fig. 1) occupying the middle of the nasal cavity, which on probing or suction is nontender and bleeds on touch and it seems to be coming from lateral wall as the probe could be passed around its medial, inferior and superior surface of mass. Nasal septum is not affected and there is mild deviation towards the opposite, i.e. left side.

    Posterior rhinoscopy is done to detect any growth in the choana or nasophaynx.

4. Palatal (oral) or inferior surface is examined which includes gingivolabial sulcus, teeth and gums, hard and soft palate. Normally, gingivolabial sulcus is examined first by inspection and then by

palpation with finger after wearing gloves. Normally, gingivolabial sulcus is not full, not obliterated, not tender and overlay mucosa is healthy, smooth and not adherent. Its involvement may show obliteration of sulcus, tenderness is present, mucosa may be discolored with loss of normal shining and become adherent. Teeth and gums are examined completely and thoroughly, note tenderness, looseness, or absence. In case of absence or with history of extraction, the socket is examined for presence of granulation tissues pus or for any evidence of antral fistula. Hard palate is looked for any fullness, swelling, ulcer or fistula and comparing with opposite half. Soft palate is examined for any swelling, ulcer and restricted mobility or paralysis.

5. The posterior surface of the maxilla cannot be directly examined. If the posterior surface is involved, tumor spreads into pterygomaxillary fossa and then sphenopalatine ganglion and maxillary nerve is involved. So there may be loss of cheek sensation (due to maxillary nerve involvement into the sphenopalatine fossa or due to inferior orbital nerve involvement in the antrum at its canal) or there may be lacrimation due to involvement of sphenopalatine ganglion or vidian nerve by affecting the parasynthetic fibers to lacrimal glands. Similarly, the pterygoid muscles may also be infiltrated by growth on posterior extension, causing trismus. Thus, these are indirect evidence of extension of maxillary antral lesion across the posterior wall. In the present case, two surfaces superficial and nasal are involved. The mass is friable and bleeds on tough, favors a diagnosis of malignant nature.

Q.3 What is the incidence of neoplasm of nose and paranasal sinuses?
Ans. It is very rare and constitutes only 0.5% of head and neck malignancy. In nasal cavity 50% are benign and 50% are malignant. In paranasal sinuses malignant are common.

Q.4 What are various locations of tumor?
Ans. 1. Maxillary sinus—70%.
2. Ethmoidal—20%.
3. Sphenoid—3%.
4. Frontal—1%.

Q.5 What are various etiological factors?
Ans. These are common between 50 and 70-year-old males, with male to female ratio 2:1.
Predisposing factors are:
1. Nickle workers are at risk for squamous cell carcinoma (100 to 870 times) may develop after 10 or more years of exposure and after 20 years of latency.
2. Wood workers for adenocarcinoma (Ethmoidal sinus).
3. Leather shoe workers for adenocarcinoma.
4. Industrial fumes, leather tanning.
5. Inhalants like chronic pigment, radium paint, mustard gas and hydrocarbons.

6. Alcohol consumption and manufacturers.
7. Tobacco has no much association with sinonasal carcinoma.

Q.6 Which group of malignant tumor is common?

Ans. A diverse group of malignant tumor can occur. Squamous cell carcinoma—70%; Adenocarcinoma—10%; Adenoid cystic carcinoma—10%; Other miscellaneous—10%.

Q.7 How does maxillary cancer present?

Ans. Carcinoma of the maxilla may present with some or all features:
   1. Oral symptoms (25–35%): Pain, trismus, alveolar ridge fullness, erosion.
   2. Nasal symptoms (50%): Nasal obstruction, epistaxis, nasal discharge.
   3. Ocular features (25%): Epiphora, diplopia, proptosis.
   4. Facial signs: Paresthesia, asymmetry, swelling.
   5. Cervical signs (10%): Metastatic neck lymph nodes especially submandibular region.

Q.8 What are various investigations?

Ans. Investigations are:
   1. CT scan and/or MRI.
   2. Endoscopy and biopsy.
   3. FNAC if cervical metastasis.
   4. PET: Can be helpful to regional and distant metastasis detection.

Q.9 What is TNM staging of sinonasal malignancy?

A.   The N and M categories are same as elsewhere.
     Maxillary sinus: Primary Tumor (T).
   T0:   No evidence of primary tumor.
   TX: Minimum requirements to assess the primary tumor cannot be met.
         T is carcinoma in situ.
   T1:   Tumor limited to antral mucosa.
   T2:   Tumor causing erosion or destruction into hard palate or lateral nasal wall (middle meatus).
   T3:   Tumor eroding posterior wall or subcutaneous or cheek or inferior or medial orbit, anterior ethmoidal sinus.
   T4:   Intracranial extension or orbital apex or skin of nose, posterior ethmoid, sphenoid, nasopharynx, soft palate, base of skull, pterygopalatine fossa, infratemporal fossa.
     Ethmoidal sinus:
   T1:   Confined to ethmoid.
   T2:   Extends to nasal cavity.
   T3:   Extends to anterior orbit or maxillary antrum.
   T4:   Intracranial extension.

Q.10 What is the prognosis of sinonasal malignancy?

Ans. Prognosis is poor with less than 50% of patients surviving for 5 years.

Q.11 What are various benign tumors of the nose?
Ans. Benign tumors of the nose and sinuses are:
1. Papilloma.
2. Inverted papilloma (4%) of sino nasal tumor.
3. Osteomas.
4. Fibrous dysplasia.
5. Neurogenic tumor.
6. Odontogenic tumors.

Q.12 What are the salient features of inverted papilloma?
Ans. It is also called Ringterz's tumor, transitional cell papilloma.
1. These constitute 4% of sinonasal tumors.
2. These arise from lateral wall.
3. These arise mostly unilateraly may extend posteriorly hanging down in the nasopharynx (only 2% bilateral).
4. Malignant degeneration occurs in 2–13%. High risk of recurrence following surgery.
5. Transnasal resection (50–80% recurrence)
6. Medial maxillectomy (lateral rhinotomy) 10–20% recurrence.
7. Endoscopic medial maxillectomy (10–20% recurrence).

Q.13 What is the importance of definite surgery in inverted papilloma?
Ans. If tumor is simply excised, it may recur aggressively with bony destruction and intracranial extension (27–73%) and may transform to malignancy (10–15%).

Q.14 What are various malignant tumors of the nose and sinuses?
Ans. 1. Squamous cell carcinoma: Most common.
     Maxillary antrum—70%; Nasal cavity—20%.
2. Adenocarcinoma: Common in superior portion.
3. Adenoid cystic carcinoma: It can spread perineural, recurrence common, neck lymph node rare.
4. Mucoepidermoid tumor.
5. Olfactory neuroblastoma: Arises from stem cells of neural crest differentiating into olfactory sensory cells.
6. Sarcoma: Osteogenic sarcoma, fibrosacroma, chondrosarcoma, rhabdomyosarcoma.
7. Lymphoma.
8. Metastatic tumor.
9. Sinonasal undiffentiated carcinoma.

Q.15 What are the earliest suspicion features of sinonasal malignancy?
Ans. 1. Unexplained epistaxis.
2. Unexplained ephiphora.
3. Dental neuralgia.
4. Non-healing socket.
5. Frequent change of dental contour or denture.
6. Flattening of dental arch.

7. Submandibular lymph node.
8. Diplopia.

Q.16 What are common classification of paranasal sinus tumors?
Ans. 1. Ohngren's classification.
2. Lederman's classifcation.
3. TNM.
4. Harrison.
5. Sisson's.

Q.17 What is Ohngren's classification?
Ans. An imaginary oblique line extending from the medial canthus of the eye to the angle of mandible and a second line passing vertically through the pupil. Tumors posterior to these lines are dangerous when compared to anterior tumors and have a poor prognosis because of their tendency to spread superiorly and posteriorly. Tumor below the line is more easily resected.

Q.18 What is Lederman's classification?
Ans. 1. Two horizontal lines passing through floor of the orbit and floor of the nasal cavity divided into three region like supra-, meso- and infra-structure (Fig. 4).
2. Two vertical lines passing through medial orbital margin again divided each region in three (middle, right and left), thus a total nine segments are formed.

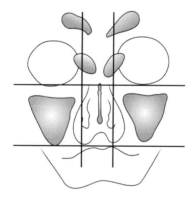

Fig. 4: Lederman's classification

Q.19 What is staging of tumor?
Ans. Staging of tumor is as follows:

Stage I	:	Tl	N0	M0			
Stage II	:	T2	N0	M0			
Stage III	:	T3	N0	M0	or		
		Tl	or	T2	or	T3	
Stage IV-A	:	T4	N0	M0	T4	Nl	M0
- B	:	Tl-T4	N2	M0	or		
		Tl-T4	N3				
- C	:	T2-T4	N1-N3	Ml			

Whenever lymph node metastasis occurs minimum stage III malignancy is present.

Q.20 What investigations are to be done?
Ans. 1. X-ray of PNS Water's view, Caldwell's view, lateral view, base of skull i.e. axial view (Hurst's view).
2. CT Scan.
3. MRI.

Q.21 What is the line of Baclesse in X-ray base of skull?
Ans. It is a part of S-shaped line and represent posterior wall of maxillary antrum. Its invasion means spread to sphenopalatine fossa.

Q.22 What is the treatment for maxillary carcinoma?
Ans. Surgery can be curative if resection is complete. Postoperative radiotherapy: is given for—
1. Large tumor.
2. Positive margins.
3. Perineural or perivascular invasion.
4. Lymph node metastasis.

Q.23 What are various hazards of radiotherapy in maxillary region?
Ans. 1. 100% of eyes receiving 5800 rads develop severe panophthalmopathy with severe corneal ulceration.
2. 86% of eye receiving 2800–5400 rads develop cataracts and visual disturbances.

Q.24 What is the role of radical neck dissection?
Ans. When metastasis is present in neck nodes, maxillectomy is done along with block dissection of neck on that side.

Q.25 What are the contraindications for surgery?
Ans. 1. Distant metastasis.
2. Inoperable metastastic nodes.
3. Involvement of the base of skull.
4. Involvement of nasopharyngeal structures.
5. Spread of growth beyond midline.

Q.26 If a growth of maxilla in advanced stage causes lesion in the nose, palate and face, from which part should a biopsy be taken?
Ans. From nasal cavity growth, because it is unexposed area and bleeding can be controlled by nasal packing.

Q.27 What does cervical metastasis in neck in case of malignancy maxilla signify?
Ans. Growth has extended to nose or overlying skin, palate or alveolus, and nasopharynx.

Q.28 Which anatomical site for carcinoma of maxillary sinus has good prognosis and is least harmful according to Ohngren's classification?
Ans. Anteroinferior medial site.

Q.29 What are various surgical approaches?

Ans. These are:

1. Endoscopic.
2. Lateral rhinotomy.
3. Transoral/transpalatel.
4. Midfacial degloving.
5. Weber Fergusson.
6. Combined craniofacial approach.
7. Trotter's incision for partial maxillectomy (small limited tumor).

Q.30 What are various maxillectomy?

Ans. These are:

1. Medial maxillectomy.
2. Inferior maxillectomy.
3. Total maxillectomy.
4. Radical maxillectomy.
5. Extended maxillectomy.

Q.31 What is radical maxillectomy?

Ans. Orbital exenteration with maxilla.

Q.32 What are the indications for orbital exenteration?

Ans. Indications are:

1. Involvement of the orbital apex.
2. Involvement of the extraocular muscles.
3. Involvement of the bulbar conjunctiva or sclera.
4. Lid involvement beyond a reasonable hope for reconstruction.
5. Nonresectable full-thickness invasion through the periorbita into the retrobulbar fat.

Q.33 What are the criteria for unresectable tumor?

Ans. 1. Tumor with superior extension into frontal lobe.
2. Lateral extension into cavernous sinus.
3. Posterior extension into prevertebral fascia and bilateral optic nerve involvement.

Q.34 How does ethmoidal sinus tumor present?

Ans. Symptoms are usually present when the ethmoid sinus tumor, spreads into vital structures like orbit, maxillary sinus, sphenoid sinus and anterior cranial fossa. Symptoms are unilateral nasal obstruction, severe headache and diplopia.

Q.35 How does sphenoid sinus tumors present?

Ans. Sphenoid sinus lies between the carotid arteries and just inferior and anterior to the optic chiasma and pituitary gland. Invasion of skull base occurs in about 50% of cases. The symptoms are headache, diplopia or loss of vision.

Q.36 How does nasal tumor present?

Ans. Presentation depends on site of origin and spread and extension of adjoining space and invasion of structures. Nasal tumor presents with nasal obstruction, rhinorrhea, epistaxis and features of sinusitis.

Q.37 Where does sinonasal tumors metastasize?

Ans. First metastasis occurs in retropharyngeal node and/or subsequently in submandibular lymph nodes. Cervical metastasis at the time of presentation is 10%, but eventually it increases to 44%.

Q.38 What is anatomy of sphenopalatine fossa?

Ans. It is also called pterygopalatine fossa. It is a small pyramidal space behind the posterior wall of maxilla below the apex of the orbit. It is bounded above by posterior surface of maxilla; posteriorly lies the root of pterygoid process and anterior surface of greater wing of sphenoid; medially by perpendicular plate of ethmoid and orbital process of palatine bone; superiorly by body of sphenoid; inferiorly the space is closed by pyramidal process of palatine bone. Contents are:

1. Maxillary nerve and its branches, i.e. zygomatic and posterior alveolar.
2. Sphenopalatine ganglion and vidian nerve.
3. Third part of internal maxillary artery and its branches.
4. Pterygoid muscles.

It communicates with

1. Orbit through inferior orbital fossa.
2. Middle cranial fossa through foramen rotundum.
3. Nasal cavity by sphenopalatine foramen.
4. Infratemporal fossa by pterygomaxillary fissure.

Q.39 What is the significance of spread of cancer to sphenopalatine fossa.

Ans. 1. Involvement of pterygoid muscle causing trismus.
2. Sphenopalatine ganglion invasion causing decreased lacrimation.

Q.40 What are the anatomical features of infratemporal fossa?

Ans. It is a space bounded superiorly by infratemporal surface of greater wing of sphenoid and small part of squamous temporal bone. Inferiorly it is open.

Medial wall is formed by lateral pterygoid palate and the pyramidal process of the palatine bone and lateral wall is formed by ramous of the mandible. Anterior wall is formed by the posterior surface of maxilla and medial surface of zygomatic bone. Contents of infratemporal fossa are;

1. Arteries: First and second part of the maxillary artery and their branches are posterior superior alveolar branch of third part.
2. Veins: Pterygoid venous plexus and maxillary vein.
3. Nerves: Mandibular nerve, chorda tympani part of maxillary nerve and posterior superior alveolar nerve.
4. Muscles: Lateral and medial pterygoid muscles, temporalis (lower part) and buccinator (lower part).

Index

Page numbers followed by *f* refer to figure